MONOCYTES, MONOCYTOSIS

AND

MONOCYTIC LEUKEMIA

Monocytes, Monocytosis and Monocytic Leukemia

By

LAWRENCE KASS, M.S., M.D.

Associate Professor of Internal Medicine
Research Associate, The Thomas Henry Simpson
Memorial Institute for Medical Research
The University of Michigan, Ann Arbor, Michigan

and

BERTRAM SCHNITZER, M.D.

Associate Professor of Pathology
The University of Michigan, Ann Arbor, Michigan

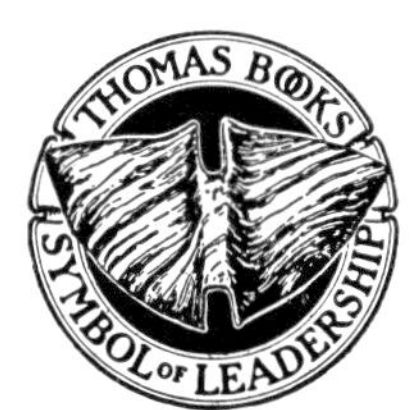

CHARLES C THOMAS • PUBLISHER
Springfield • Illinois • USA

Published and Distributed Throughout the World by
CHARLES C THOMAS • PUBLISHER
Bannerstone House
301–327 East Lawrence Avenue, Springfield, Illinois, U.S.A.

© *1973, by* CHARLES C THOMAS • PUBLISHER
ISBN 0-398—02883-4
Library of Congress Catalog Card Number: 73-5932

Library of Congress Cataloging in Publication Data

Kass, Lawrence.
   Monocytes, monocytosis, and monocytic leukemia.

   Bibliography: p.
   1. Monocytes. 2. Monocytic leukemia.
I. Schnitzer, Bertram, joint author. II. Title.
[DNLM: 1. Leukemia, Monocytic. 2. Monocytes.
WH 200 K18m 1973]
RC643.K37   616.1'5   73-5932
ISBN 0-398-02883-4

Printed in the United States of America
CC-1

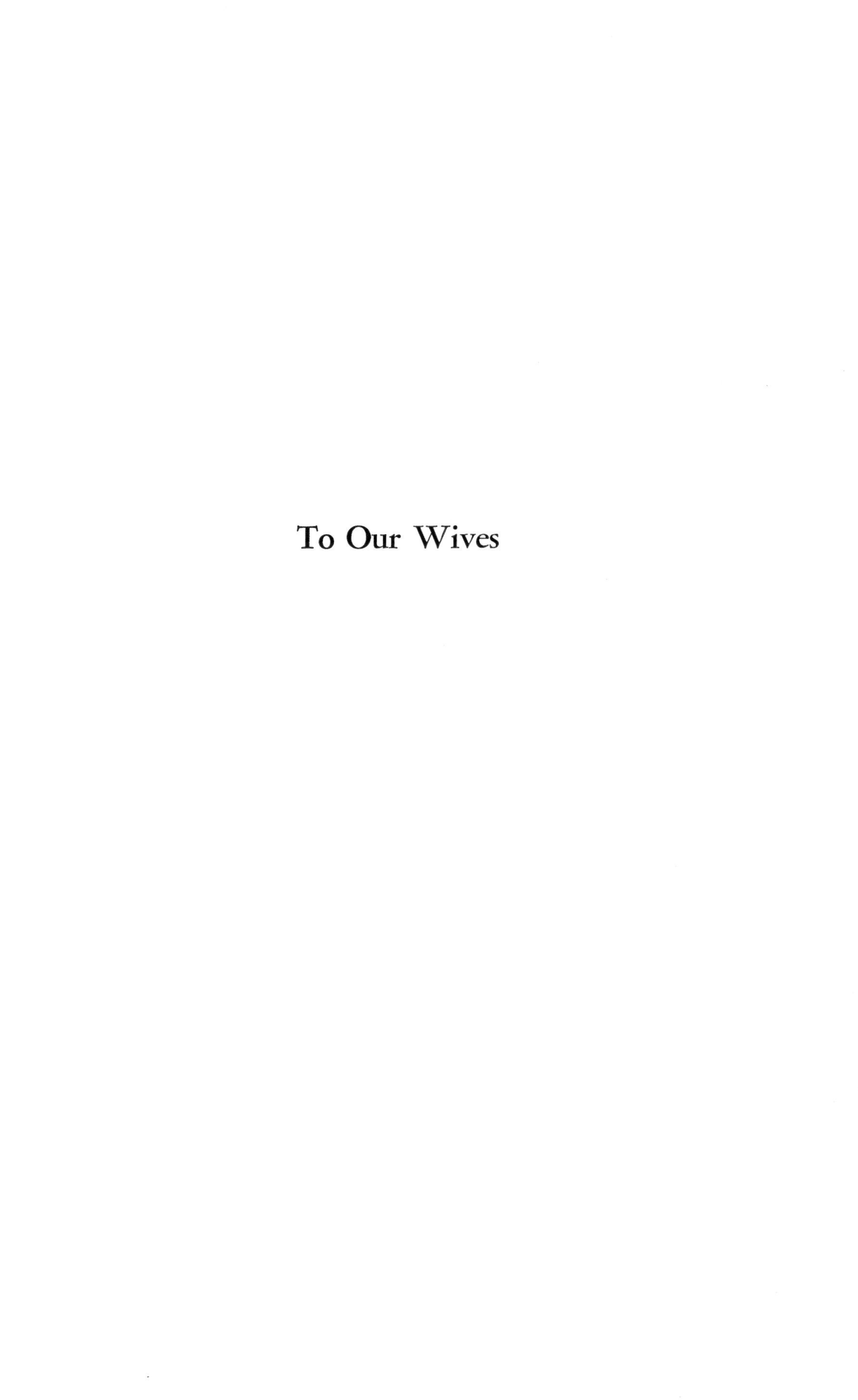

To Our Wives

PREFACE

THIS IS A BOOK about the monocyte and about conditions in which increased numbers of either benign or neoplastic monocytes can be found. It has been written for hematologists, pathologists, oncologists and immunologists because interest in the monocyte spans all of these disciplines to a remarkable degree.

Among blood cells, the monocyte is unique in its ability to assume different morphologic appearances and functions in diverse situations. Indeed, it is the cell "of a thousand faces."

This monograph intentionally avoids the polemicism characteristic of the early part of the twentieth century, an era where heated debates as to the origin and potentialities of the monocyte were frequent. Some of these aspects of the monocyte are still matters of controversy.

We wish to thank Drs. C. J. D. Zarafonetis and Muriel C. Meyers for reviewing the manuscript and providing valuable suggestions. Dr. Meyers provided the photographs illustrating gingival and dermatologic manifestations of monocytic leukemia. We also appreciate the expert technical assistance of Robert D. Farnsworth and Michael L. Mead, and thank Barbara A. Stoner and Barbara Walentowski for secretarial assistance.

We hope that the various criteria for the diagnosis of the disorders of monocytes will be amplified and clarified by the considerations raised in this book. It is our intent that the material presented here will serve to incite greater interest in an important yet elusive cell.

This work was supported in part by the Elizabeth Roodvoets Memorial Grant for Cancer Research of the American Cancer Society (CI-79) and by a grant from the National Cancer Institute (USPH CA 14428-01).

LAWRENCE KASS
BERTRAM SCHNITZER

CONTENTS

MONOCYTES, MONOCYTOSIS

AND

MONOCYTIC LEUKEMIA

CHAPTER I

HISTORICAL ASPECTS OF MONOCYTES

I N 1879 PAUL EHRLICH (Fig. 1) described differences in the staining properties of leukocyte granules. (84)   In 1880 (85) on the basis of

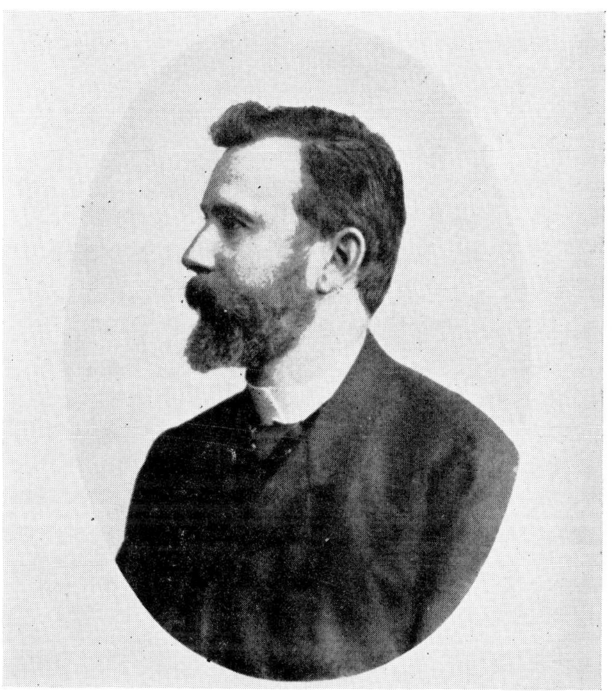

Figure 1. Paul Ehrlich (from Gallerie hervorragender Aertze und Naturforscher. *Muench Med Wochensch 61·575, 1915.* Reprinted with permission of J. F. Lehmanns Verlag).

these staining differences, he was able to separate leukocytes into two groups, "polynuclear and mononuclear." Ehrlich states:

As mentioned already, not all lymphocytes contain Σ (neutrophilic) granulation; there are always some cells that do not contain granulation and which differ also with regard to their morphological and microchemical characteristic. The cells which contain granulation usually show peculiar polymorphogenic types of nuclei or several small round and heavily stained nuclei. The smaller group of cells shows elements that contain a large plump, ovoid and poorly stained nucleus and a relatively small amount of protoplasm. . . *Especially in the leuko-cythemic blood there are often cells which show sparse Σ granulation and which—according to their appearance—take a position between the types of cells . . . described above.*

In his *Lectures on the Comparative Pathology of Inflammation* in 1891, Metchnikoff (186) traced the development of mononuclear phagocytes through various forms of invertebrate and vertebrate life. As illustrated in Plate 1, Metchnikoff described the phagocytic capacity of these cells and postulated that they were related phylogenetically to unicellular organisms such as the amoeba. Cells which we might consider monocytes were then called "large mononuclear leukocytes." Metchnikoff believed that these cells had unique cytoplasmic and nuclear properties and differed from normal lymphocytes in that they were larger and had an oval, bean or kidney-shaped nucleus.

In 1892 Ehrlich and Lazarus (86) stated that "large mononuclear cells" in the blood change into

. . . the *transitional forms*. These resemble the preceding but are distinguished by deep notches in the nucleus, which often give it an hour-glass shape, further by a somewhat greater affinity for stains, and by the presence of scanty neurophil granulations in the protoplasm.

These "transitional cells" are what we now call monocytes.

In pathological specimens obtained from patients with typhoid fever, Mallory (161) in 1898 traced the origin of the monocyte (mononuclear phagocyte) to endothelial cells of blood vessels. Using rabbit omentum and vital stains, Ranvier (216) in 1899 described what he called "clasmatocytes." These were large histiocytic cells with dendritic processes and a capacity to ingest vital stains.

In 1900 Otto Naegeli described the morphological characteristics of the myeloblast. (195) Naegeli held the view that the myeloblast was the precursor of the monocyte. He believed that monocytic leukemia per se did not exist as a separate entity, but was rather a monocytic variant of acute myeloblastic leukemia. (196,197,198) Naegeli did not actually describe myelomonocytic leukemia (Chapter IV). It was Downey who in 1938 applied the name "Naegeli-type" monocytic leukemia to this mixed granulocytic-monocytic leukemia. (79)

In some of his early studies on inflammation in 1903 (166) and in 1927, (167) Maximow described and illustrated large mononuclear cells, apparently different from lymphocytes, that had exhibited phagocytic properties when exposed to vital dyes, and in addition could transform into fibroblasts in tissue cultures. Maximow called these cells "polyblasts" and indicated that they seemed to be derived from large circulating mononuclear cells, some of which may have been lymphocytes and others monocytes.

Pappenheim and Ferrata in 1910 (208) and Pappenheim in 1911 (209) provided detailed descriptions of the monocyte. Their studies clearly differentiated the morphological features of the monocyte from those of the lymphocyte. Reproductions of several drawings from Pappenheim and Ferrata's original treatise (208) are illustrated in Plate 2. The characteristic cytoplasmic properties of the monocyte (namely the lavender-gray, lightly granular cytoplasm) when stained with a panoptic stain are illustrated. Also described in their original papers were the nuclear characteristics of the monocyte, such as the coarsely fenestrated nuclear chromatin and the characteristic fold or indentation. Pappenheim and Ferrata introduced the concept that the monocyte could exhibit a spectrum of changes, presumably reflecting the age of the cell. Schilling-Torgau in 1912 (253) also described a large mononuclear cell (presumably the monocyte) and so-called transition forms as a "third system, relatively separated from the two cell systems," i.e. lymphatic and myeloid. Three years after the original description of the monocyte, Reschad and Schilling-Torgau in 1913 (221) described the first case of monocytic leukemia (See Chapter III).

In the early 1920's Sabin and her co-workers (58,59,243,244,245, 246,247) developed the supravital staining method for the identification of different types of leukocytes. Utilizing the neutral red and Janus green staining technique, Sabin, (243,246) Cunningham, (58,59) Simpson (274) and Forkner (97) described what they thought were distinctive features of the monocyte. These were (a) a rosette of vacuoles stained with neutral red, (b) small stick-like mitochondria stained with Janus green surrounding the vacuoles, and (c) a large mononuclear cell with an indented nucleus. They felt that the monocyte could be distinguished from the lymphocyte on the basis of these criteria, since in their studies the lymphocyte did not possess such staining properties.

In a series of papers Sabin (58,244,247) and her associates developed an additional theory of origin of the monocyte, namely from the so-called "monoblast." They were of the opinion, as was McJunkin, (172,173,174,175,176) that the monocyte had an intimate relationship to the endothelial cells of blood vessels, and they thought that, in certain situations, monocytes were actually derived from endothelial cells. Wiseman (305) also postulated that the monocyte was derived from the "monoblast."

Bloom (27) and Hall (116) seriously questioned the specificity of Sabin's supravital technique. On the basis of their own studies, Bloom and Hall felt that the lymphocyte frequently exhibited many of the supravital staining features which Sabin and her co-workers had attributed to the monocyte alone. Consequently, Bloom and Hall believed that the supravital technique could not be used to distinguish the lymphocyte from the monocyte. In a series of experiments using tissue cultures, Bloom (28) described the transformation of lymphocytes into cells which could not be distinguished from monocytes on morphological grounds, and he therefore postulated that the monocyte was derived from the lymphocyte. Maximow (168,169) held a similar view.

Early investigators interested in the relationships between monocytes and mycobacteria found that the monocytes exhibited active phagocytosis of mycobacteria in tissue cultures. On the basis of his tissue culture studies, Maximow theorized that the epitheloid cells of the tubercle were derived from the monocyte. Sabin (247) came to a similar conclusion regarding the role of the monocyte in tubercle formation.

In the late 1920's and 1930's, additional reports of what was then termed "monocytic leukemia" appeared, (23,30,43,48,49,56,65,89,97, 100,134,135,149,162,163,184,185,205,249,250,267,281,297,298,299) and various theories about the derivation of the monocyte were proposed. (42,65,99,177,210) In describing the appearance of histiocytes in the peripheral blood, Dameshek in 1931 (66) postulated that the histiocyte (macrophage) was identical to the "monoblast." He felt that the histiocyte and monocyte often "merge," and that the histiocyte could give rise to the monocyte. Naegeli (197,198) stated that the majority of "so-called monocytic leukemias" were actually monocytoses, and that monocytes were actually paramyeloblasts, derived ultimately from myeloblasts. Richter (225) also believed that the monocyte in monocytic leukemia was derived from the myeloblast, and Rinehart (227) stated that the development of hemohistioblasts into monocytes could be traced in monocytic leukemia.

During this period Schilling (251) developed what he called the "trialistic" theory of blood formation, in which he postulated that the monocyte was derived from a reticuloendothelial stem cell, distinct from the myeloblast and lymphoblast. A group of disorders that were characterized by a proliferation of neoplastic reticulum cells (91,111, 112,201,236,237,272) and called aleukemic reticulosis (67) in the American literature was also recognized. Some patients with these disorders exhibited peripheral blood manifestations of their disease in the form of monocytosis, whereas in other patients the disease appeared to have only a tissue phase. Today, we call these latter neoplasms reticulum cell sarcoma or histiocytic lymphoma. (217)

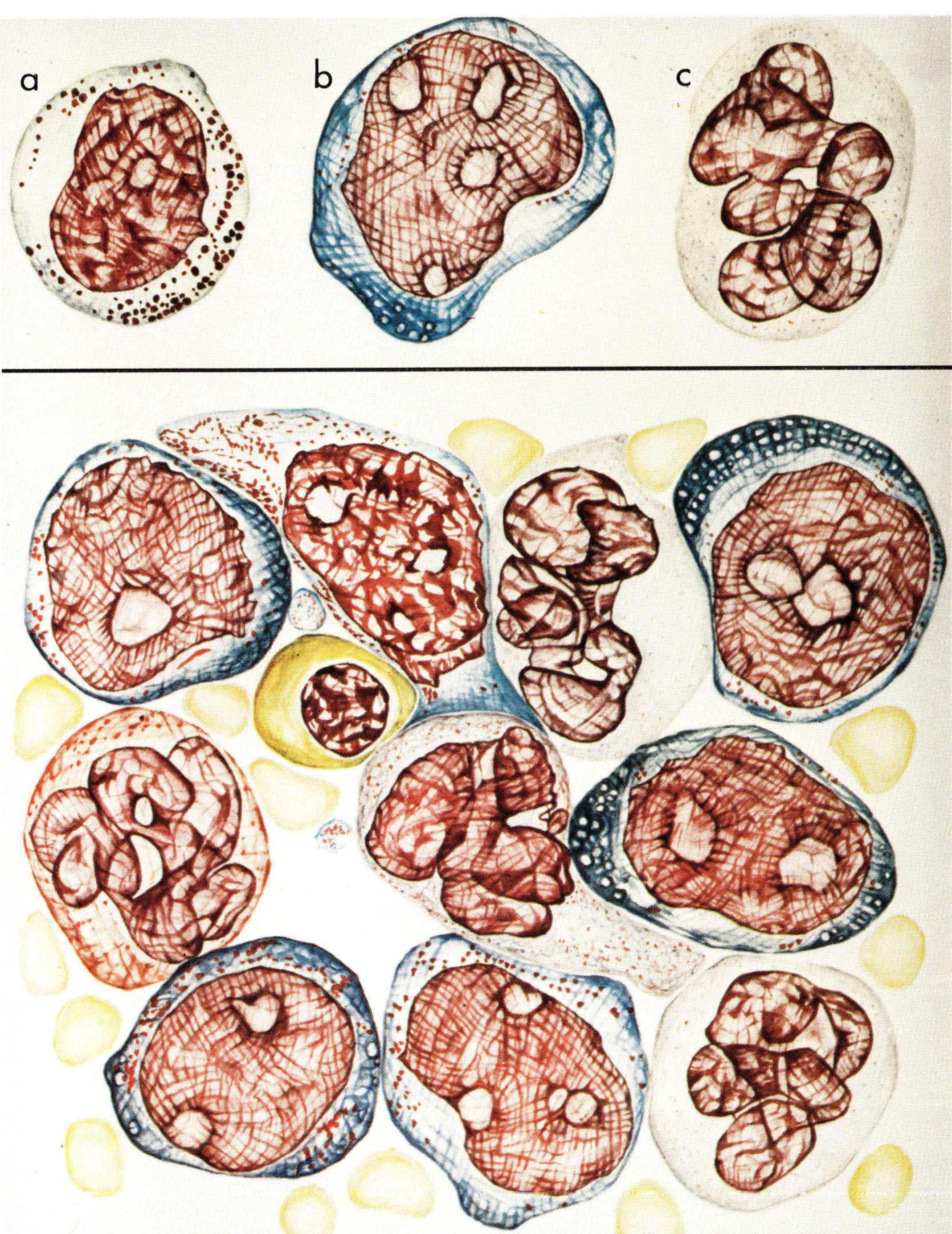

FRONTISPIECE *Acute myelomonocytic leukemia (Naegeli Type). a*-represents a progranulocyte frequently found in the peripheral blood of a patient with this disorder. *b*-is a leukemic blast, also found in the peripheral blood. Nucleoli are prominent, as is an indentation of the nucleus. Chromatin strands appear to radiate from the nucleoli. *c*-represents a neoplastic monocyte found in the peripheral blood. The nuclear lobulations appear to overlie each other in an elaborately twisted arrangement. The cytoplasm is pale lilac-colored with abundant nonspecific granules.

The grouping of cells in the lower half of the drawing represents bone marrow obtained from this same patient. Numerous leukemic blasts, some containing Auer rods, are seen. Cytoplasmic vacuoles are frequent in these blasts, as are large, prominent nucleoli. Neoplastic monocytes with elaborate foldings of their nuclei are also seen, as well as a large hemohistiocyte and a megaloblastoid intermediate macronormoblast. Some of the neoplastic monocytes have cytoplasmic "tails." (Opaque watercolor by L.K.)

Plate 1. From Metchnikoff's *Lectures on the Comparative Pathology of Inflammation* (1891). This figure illustrates phagocytosis by mononuclear cells in invertebrates (Reprinted with permission of Dover Publications.)

Plate 2. From Pappenheim and Ferrata (1911). These are early illustrations of monocytes, with their distinctive kidney-bean nuclear shape and nuclear infoldings. (Reprinted with permission of J. F. Lehmanns Verlag.)

Plate 3. (a) A normal living monocyte stained supravitally with a mixture of neutral red and Janus green. The characteristic monocyte nucleus with multiple infoldings is seen, as is abundant cytoplasm. The orange-staining *rosette* areas represent vacuoles which have been stained supravitally with neutral red. The small, green-staining objects surrounding the neutral red-staining cluster of vacuoles are mitochondria which have been stained supravitally with Janus green.

(b) A normal monocyte stained with peroxidase stain. The punctate bluish-black areas represent sites of peroxidase activity, which is greatly reduced or absent in the normal monocyte when compared to the polymorphonuclear leukocyte.

(c) Nonspecific esterase activity in the cytoplasm of a normal monocyte using alpha-napthyl acetate as substrate. The red-orange stained particulate material in the cytoplasm is the reaction product. Such areas of nonspecific esterase activity are said to be specific for the monocyte.

Plate 4. From Naegeli's *Blutkrankeiten und Blutdiagnostik* (1931). These cells are myeloblasts and monocytoid myeloblasts from the peripheral blood of a patient with acute myeloblastic leukemia. (Reprinted with permission of Julius Springer Verlag.)

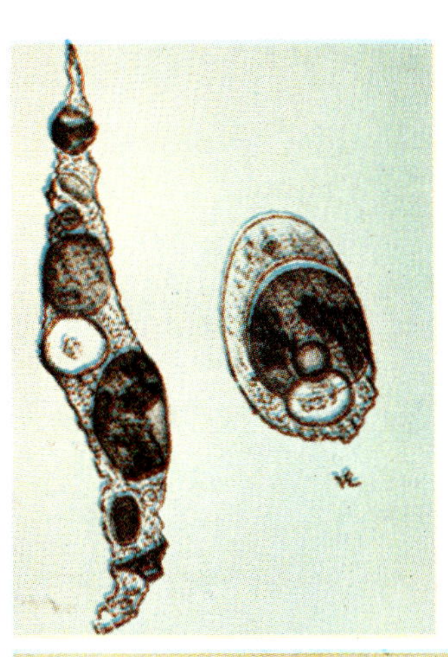

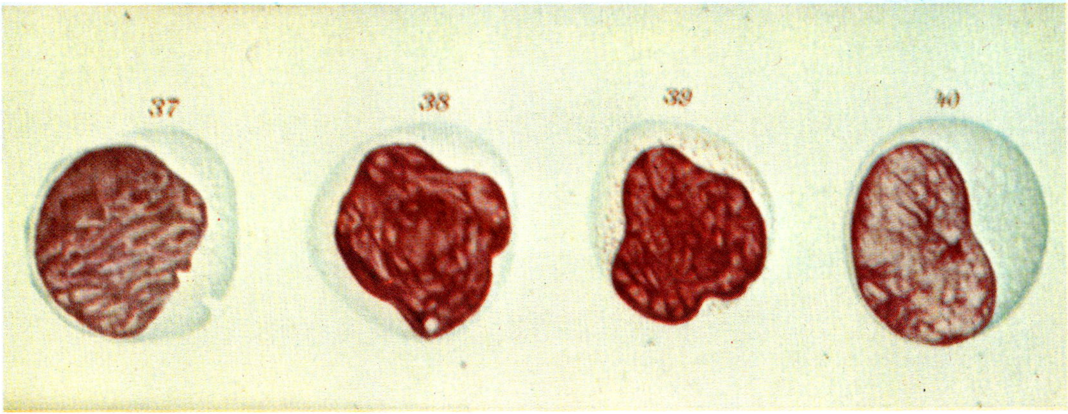

37   38   39   40

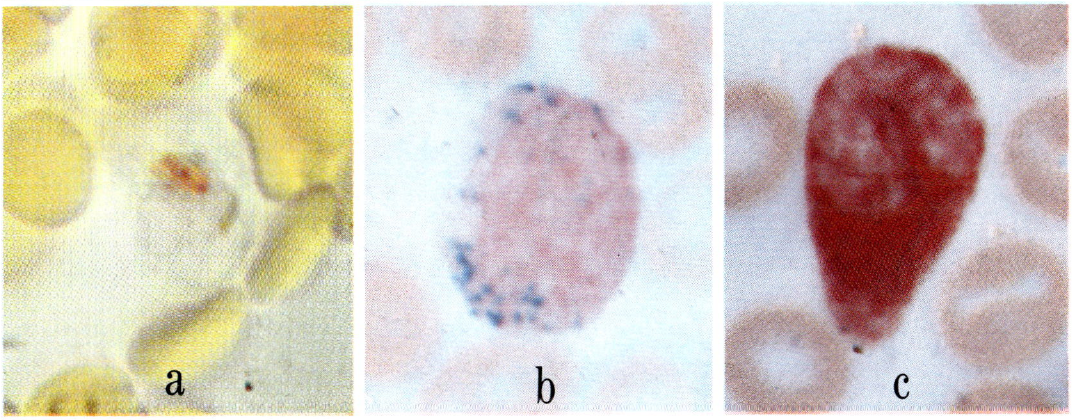

a   b   c

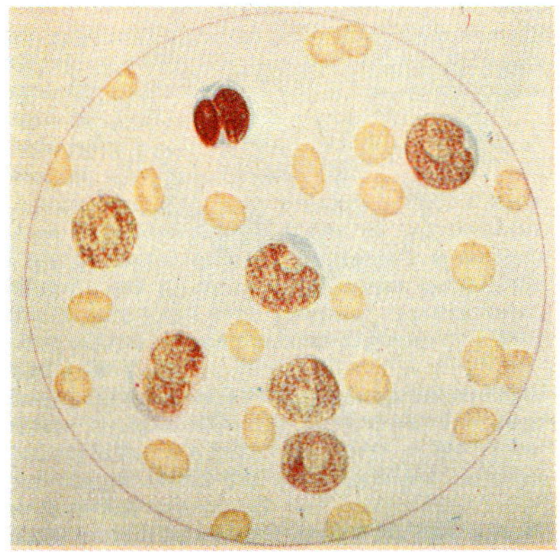

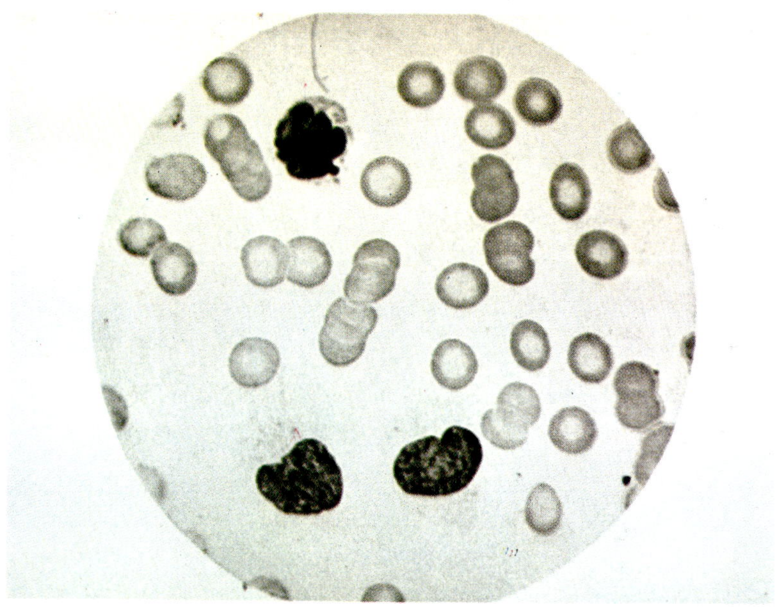

Plate 5. Monocytes from the original case of acute monocytic leukemia described in 1913 by Reschad and Schilling. (From Victor Schilling's *The Blood Picture,* translated and edited by R.B.H. Gradwohl. St. Louis, 1929. Reprinted with permission of the C.V. Mosby Co.)

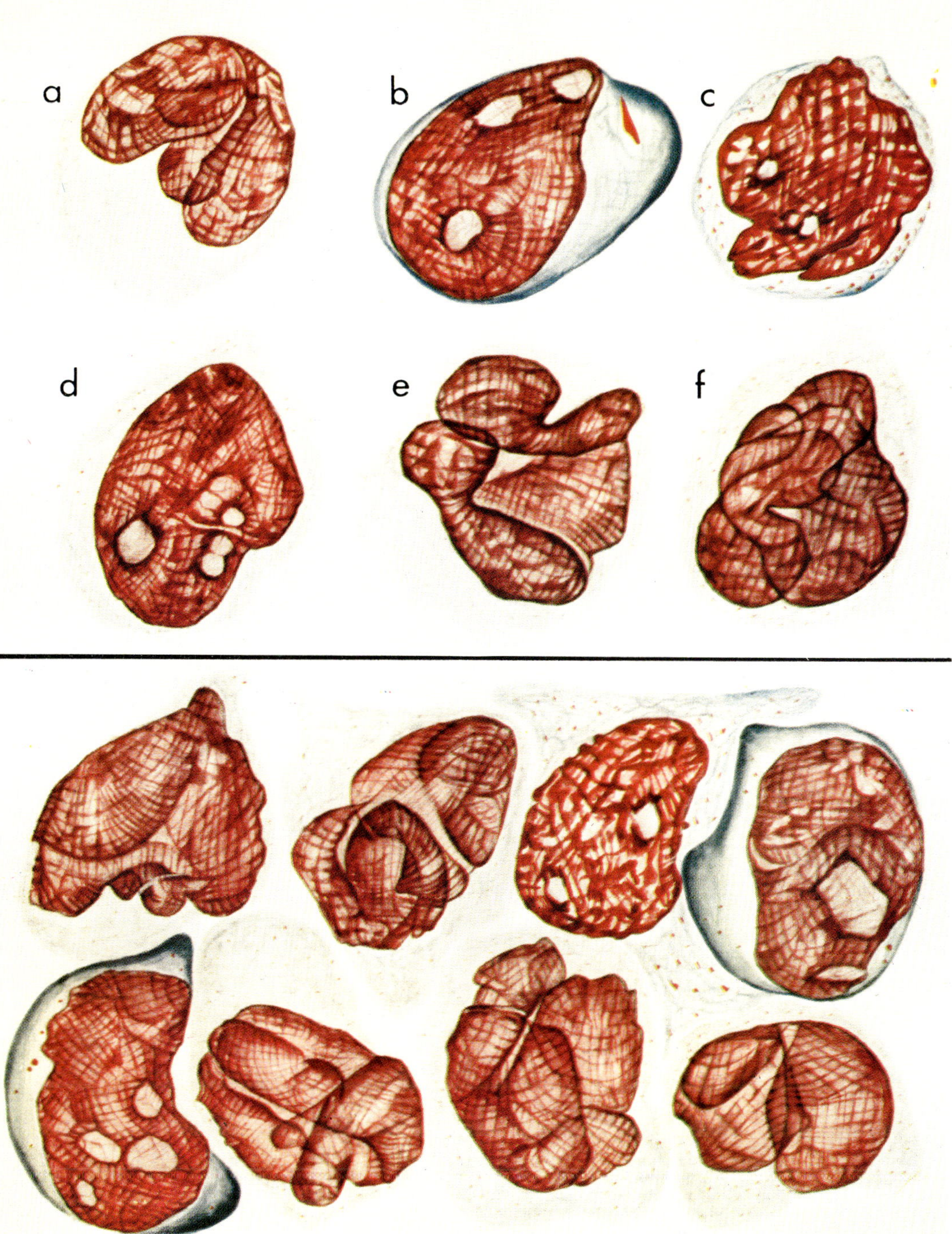

Plate 6. Acute histiomonocytic leukemia (Schilling-type). Cells *a* through *f* are monocytes found in the peripheral blood of a patient with this disorder. Cells *a, d, e* and *f* are neoplastic monocytes, with elaborately folded nuclei, delicate chromatin strands crossing each other in a web arrangement and frequent multiple nucleoli. The cytoplasm of these cells is pale lavender, with light-staining nonspecific granules. Cell *b* is a histiomonoblast with prominent nucleoli, deeply basophilic, clear cytoplasm and a large eosinophilic-staining Auer rod. *c* A hemohistioblast, a cell frequently found in the peripheral blood of patients with this disorder.

The cells in the lower half of the drawing are from the bone marrow of a patient with acute histiomonocytic leukemia. Blast cells, neoplastic monocytes with elaborate nuclear foldings and delicate chromatin, and a large hemohistioblast are found in these marrows. (Opaque watercolor by L.K.)

Plate 7. Acute histiomonocytic leukemia. In this neoplastic histiomonocyte from the peripheral blood of a patient with histiomonocytic leukemia, the nucleus shows fine chromatin which imparts a fenestrated appearance. The cytoplasm is voluminous, staining bluish-gray, and containing numerous small vacuoles and multiple pseudopodia. The nuclear features of this cell resemble those seen in a reticulum cell.

Plate 8. Circulating primitive cells from a patient with leukemic reticuloendotheliosis as illustrated by Otto Ewald in 1923. (Reprinted with permission of Julius Springer Verlag.)

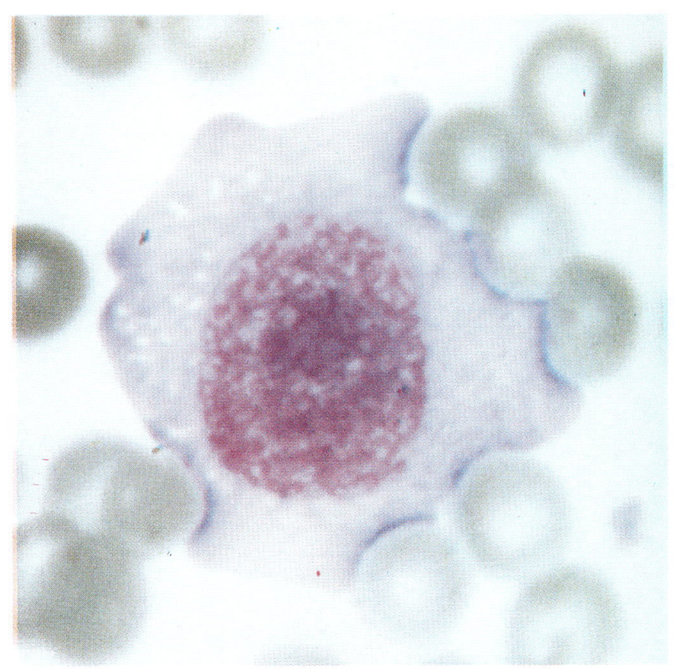

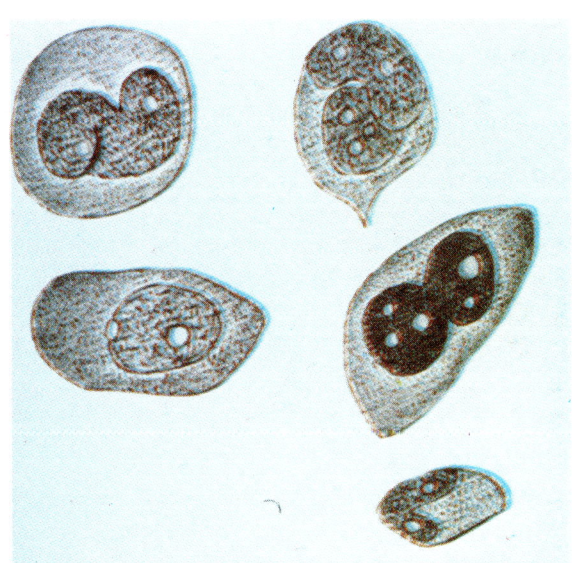

h. 1. Reticuloendothelzellen im Blutausstrich.
iß Appochromat 2 mm]1,3. Comp. Ocular 8.

Plate 9. Cells from the peripheral blood of a patient with leukemic reticuloendotheliosis. (From *Downey's Handbook of Hematology.* New York, Harper and Row, 1938, p. 1331. Reprinted with permission of Harper and Row.)

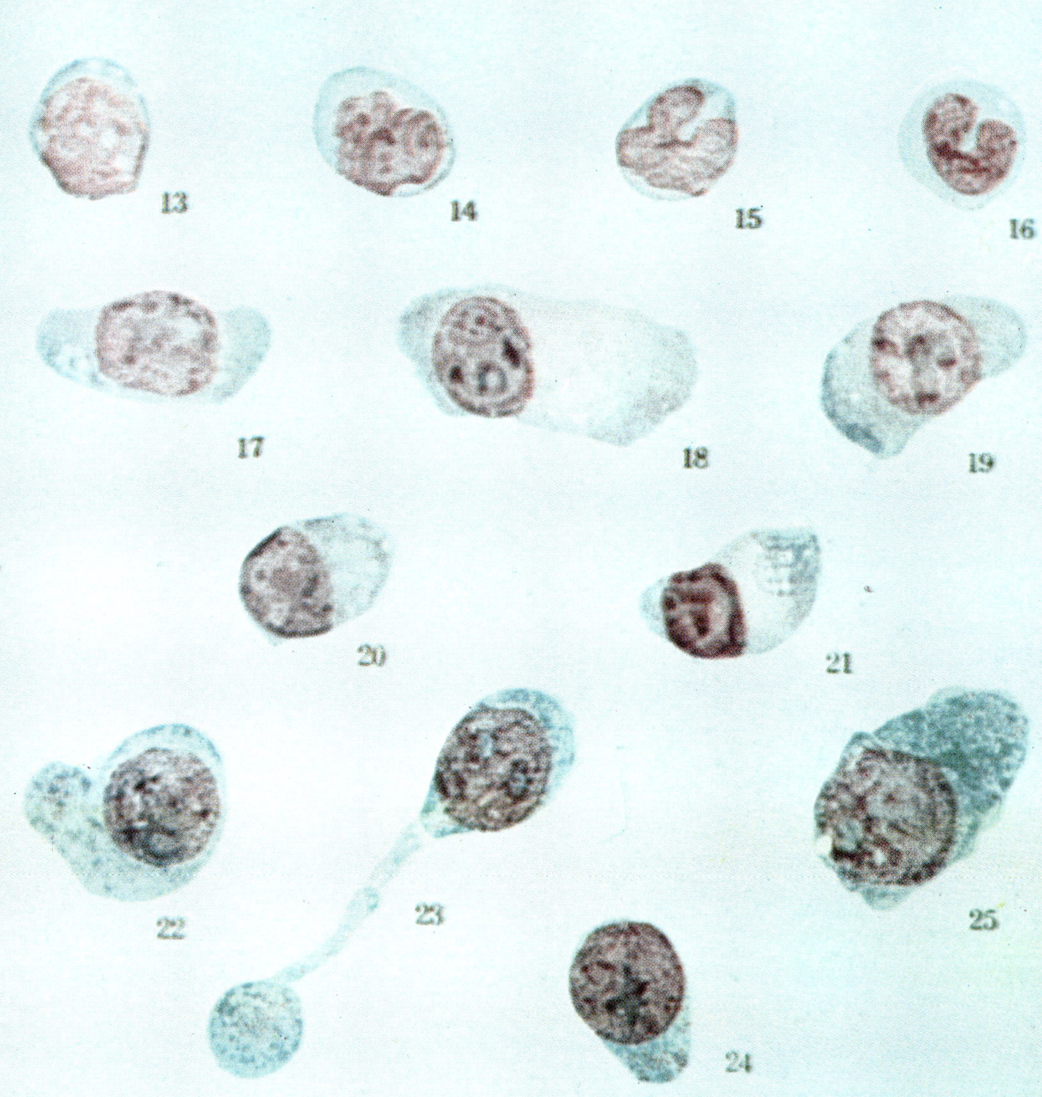
13
14
15
16
17
18
19
20
21
22
23
25
24
PLATE I

Plate 10. (a) Neoplastic reticulum cells from the bone marrow of a patient with leukemic reticulum cell sarcoma. The nuclear chromatin is fine with few or no aggregates. There are multiple prominent nucleoli surrounded by aggregated chromatin. The cytoplasm is deeply basophilic, and the cytoplasm and nuclei both contain vacuoles.

(b) The predominant cell in the peripheral blood of this patient. The chromatin is fine, and the nucleolus is unusually large with perinucleolar condensation. The cytoplasm is deeply basophilic with a striated appearance.

(c) A more monocytoid-appearing cell in the peripheral blood of this patient, appearing to be one step further in the monocytoid progression of the cell illustrated in (b). The nucleus contains several infoldings and indentations, and the cytoplasm is less basophilic and contains several vacuoles.

(d) A monocyte with aberrant-appearing nucleus in the peripheral blood of this patient. The cytoplasm stains bluish-grey, and the nucleus shows unusual segmentation and lobulation. These cells (b, c, and d) resemble those described by Downey (Plate 9).

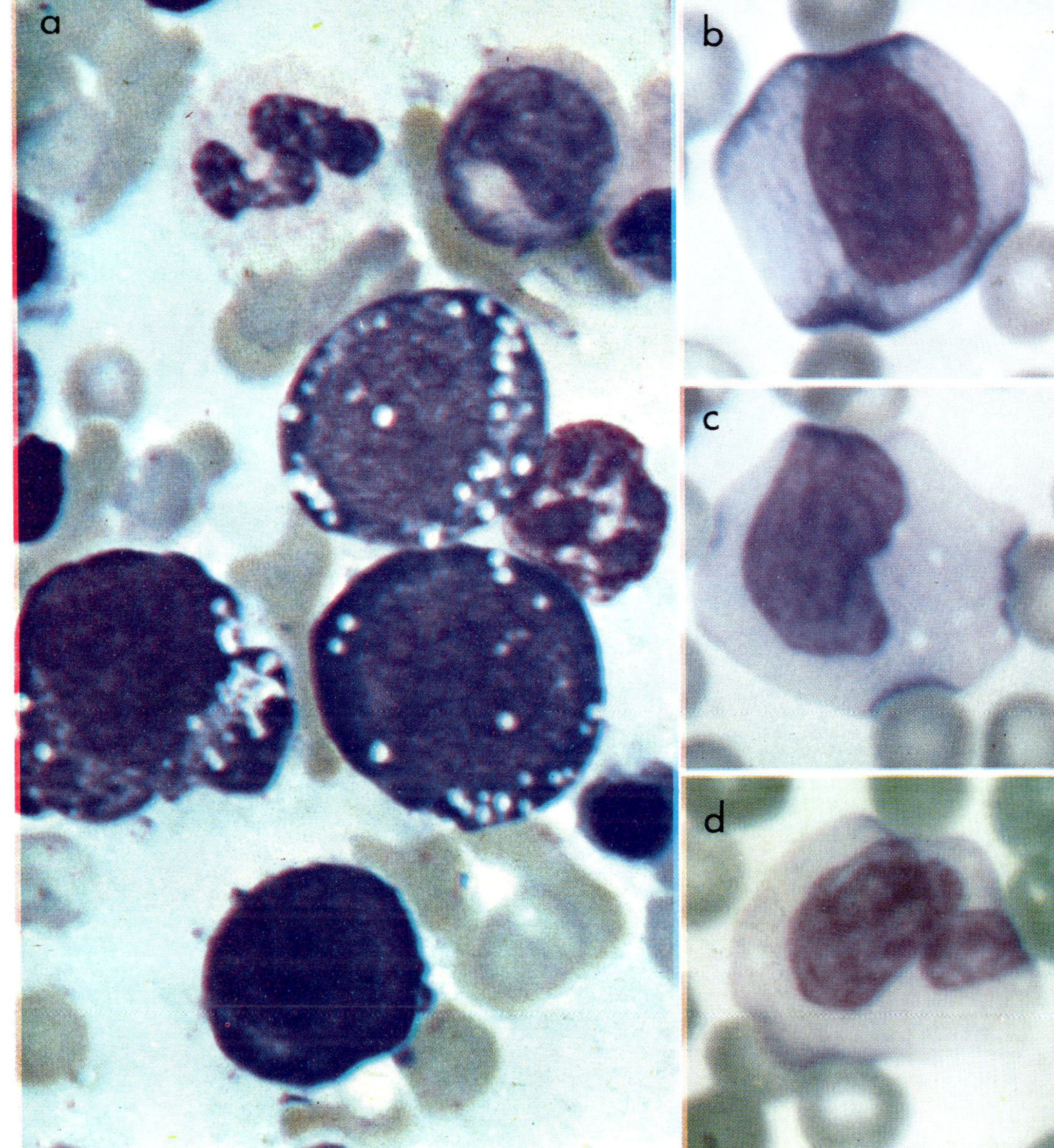

Plate 11. (a) Cells obtained from the bone marrow of this patient with leukemic reticulum cell sarcoma. Large, neoplastic-appearing monocytoid cells with multiple nuclear infoldings and lobulation are seen. Nucleoli are small. There are numerous block-like aggregates of chromatin within the nucleus. The cytoplasm is blue-gray.

(b) A neoplastic monocyte found in the peripheral blood of this patient. Numerous finger-like nuclear lobules are seen, as well as gray-lilac colored cytoplasm.

(c) Large neoplastic monocyte found in the peripheral blood of this patient. It may represent a younger form of the cell illustrated in (b). Nucleoli are present and are small. The chromatin is fine, with numerous sharply defined aggregates. The cytoplasm is blue-gray.

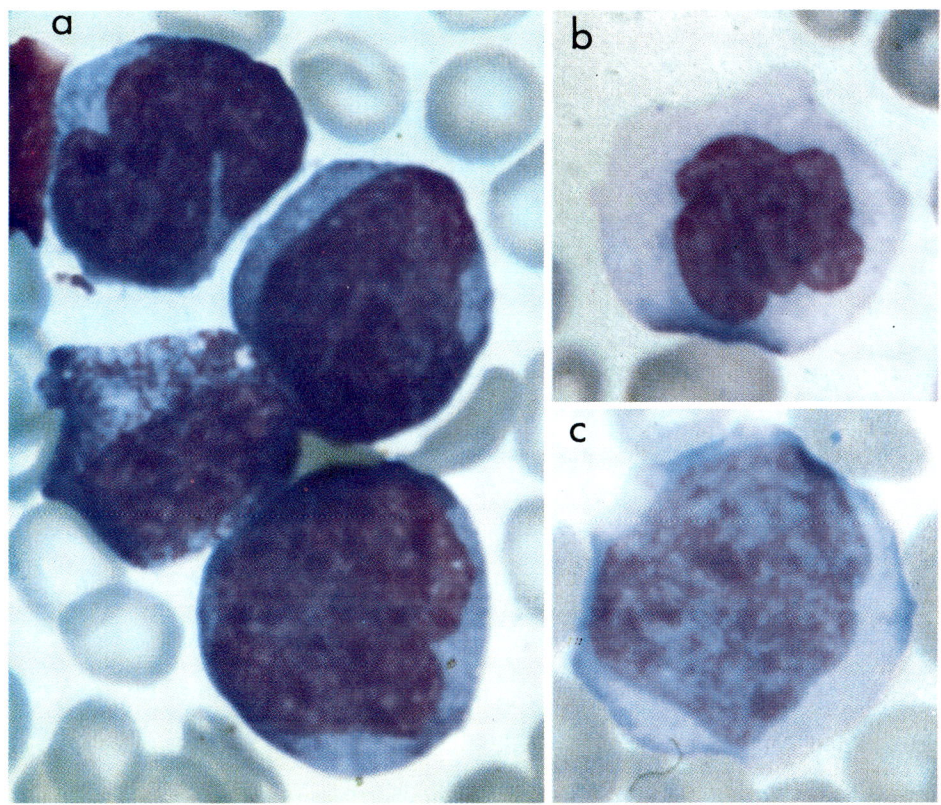

Plate 12. (a) Neoplastic histiomonocytes from the bone marrow of a patient with leukemic reticulum cell sarcoma. The nuclear chromatin is fine, and the nucleoli are prominent. The cytoplasm stains blue-gray. Cytoplasmic tails and cytoplasmic shedding are evident.

(b) A histiomonoblast found in the peripheral blood of this patient. The nuclear chromatin is fine, and there is a prominent nucleolus. The cytoplasm is deeply basophilic, with a sprinkling of nonspecific granules and several vacuoles. A cytoplasmic tail is evident.

(c) A histiomonocyte from the peripheral blood of this patient. The nucleus shows monocytoid features, with a deep indentation and lobulations. The cytoplasm is voluminous and contains numerous vacuoles of varying size, some of which are confluent. Pseudopodia are also seen.

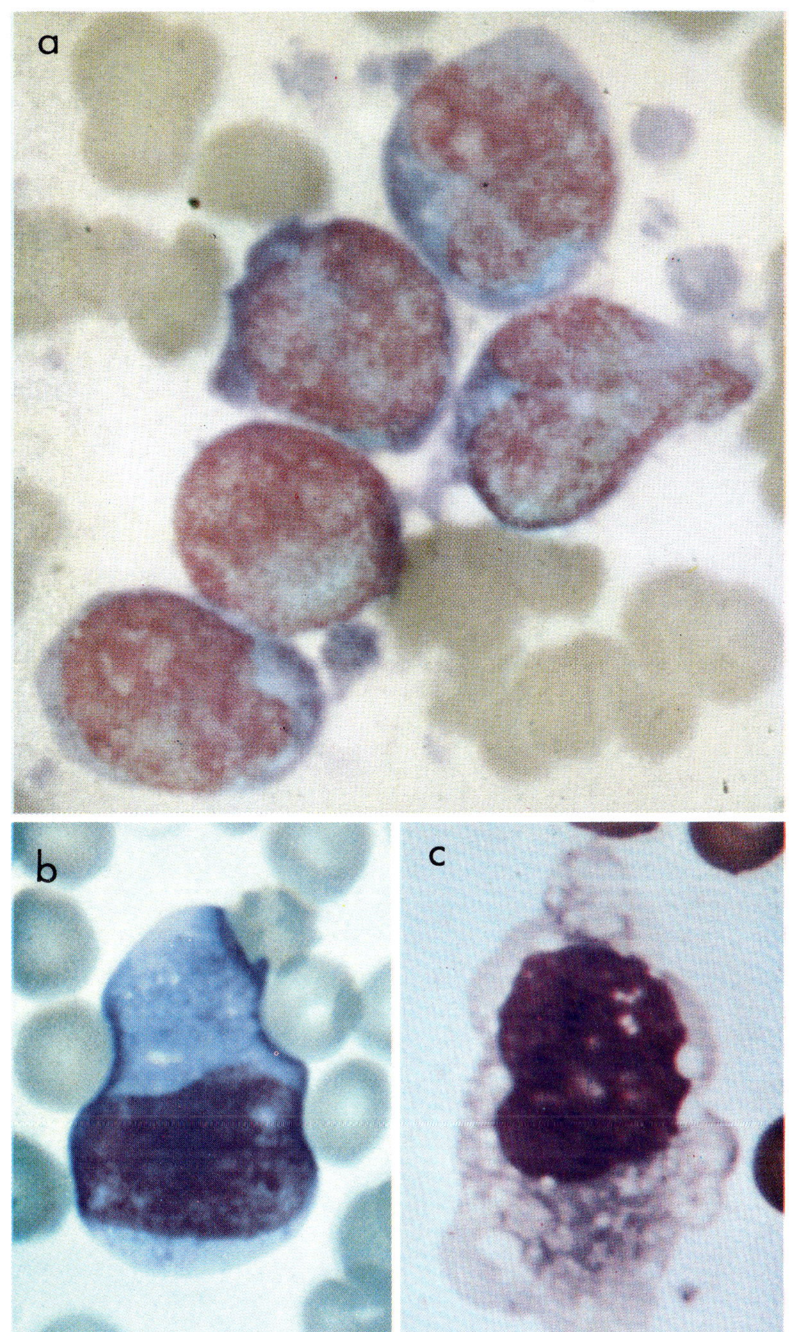

In 1938, Downey (79) expanded Ewald's concept (90) of leukemic reticuloendotheliosis, a disorder in which there were primitive neoplastic-appearing cells in the peripheral blood and in visceral organs. Cells seen in the peripheral blood and bone marrow of patients with the leukemic phase of reticulum cell sarcoma (259) closely resemble the cells from a case (Case I) of leukemic reticuloendotheliosis described and illustrated by Downey (Chapter IV).

CHAPTER II

THE NORMAL MONOCYTE

Structure

NORMAL MONOCYTES (15,38,284) in peripheral blood and bone marrow exhibit a variety of appearances, as illustrated in Figure 2. Some of these cells are *young* or primitive monocytes, since

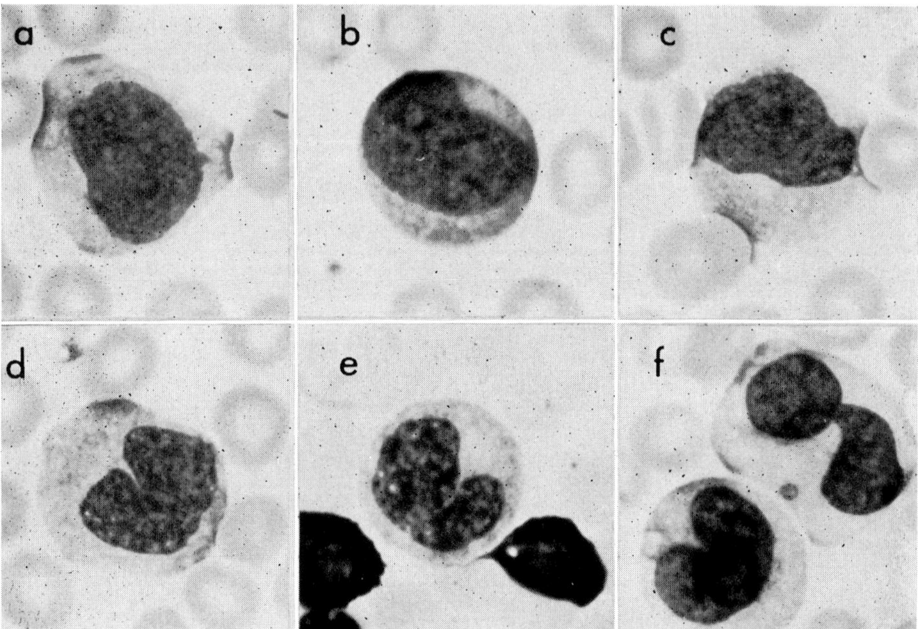

Figure 2. A spectrum of normal monocytes found in the peripheral blood (a) represents a young monocyte. The cytoplasm is lightly basophilic. The nucleus has a minimal indentation, and the nuclear chromatin is delicate and closely approximated, with little tendency toward clumping. Structures within the nucleus resemble nucleoli but may also be cellular organelles, such as the Golgi apparatus, overlying the nucleus.

(b) and (c) represent later stages of monocyte maturation. The nuclear chromatin shows a greater degree of aggregation than (a), and the cytoplasm is more lavender and contains a greater number of nonspecific granules. (d), (e) and (f) show progressive maturation of normal monocytes, with deeper indentations of the nuclei and further chromatin clumping. Actual segmentation may occur in senescent monocytes, as seen in (f).

their nucleus is large in relation to the cytoplasm, and they contain a nucleolus. As the monocyte matures, the folding or indentation in the nucleus becomes more prominent and the nucleus may exhibit lobulations. Older or senescent monocytes may have a thin, multi-lobulated nucleus which on casual inspection may resemble that of a metamyelocyte or even a polymorphonuclear leukocyte. Murthy and von Haam (194) observed that the sex chromatin in normal human monocytes occurred as a darkly staining planoconvex chromatin aggregate on the inner aspect of the nuclear membrane.

Primitive-appearing monocytoid cells which might be called "monoblasts" are very rarely seen in normal bone marrows. It is sometimes difficult to distinguish these from atypical-appearing myeloblasts. The "monoblasts" have several blocklike, somewhat angular-appearing aggregates of chromatin in the interstices of the chromatin web. The chromatin of young monocytes is somewhat finer and exhibits fewer aggregates than that of the older monocytes. When stained with a panoptic stain such as Wright's or Giemsa stain the cytoplasm of the young monocyte is slightly basophilic and opaque, in contrast to the clear blue cytoplasm of the lymphocyte. As the monocyte matures, the lilac color of the cytoplasm becomes more apparent as do the innumerable pink and azurophil granules. The cytoplasm of older or senescent monocytes may be grayish lilac. The monocyte in the Pelger-Huet anomaly is seen in Figure 3. The nuclear chromatin shows prominent blocklike aggregates, analogous to those seen in the polymorphonuclear leukocytes in this condition.

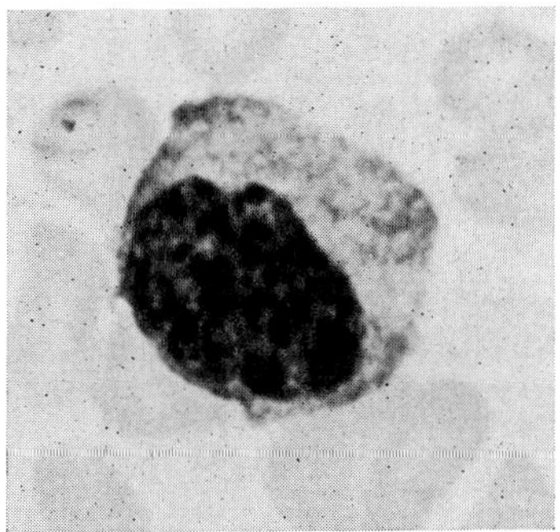

Figure 3. Monocyte from the peripheral blood of a patient with the Pelger-Huet anomaly. The nuclear chromatin of monocytes in this disorder shares aberrations found in granulocytes in the Pelger-Huet anomaly, namely sharply defined blocklike aggregates of chromatin within the nucleus.

Monocytes in sections of normal peripheral blood imbedded in Epon (Fig. 4) have large indented or horseshoe-shaped nuclei. Nucleoli are occasionally seen. The monocytes have abundant cytoplasm. The

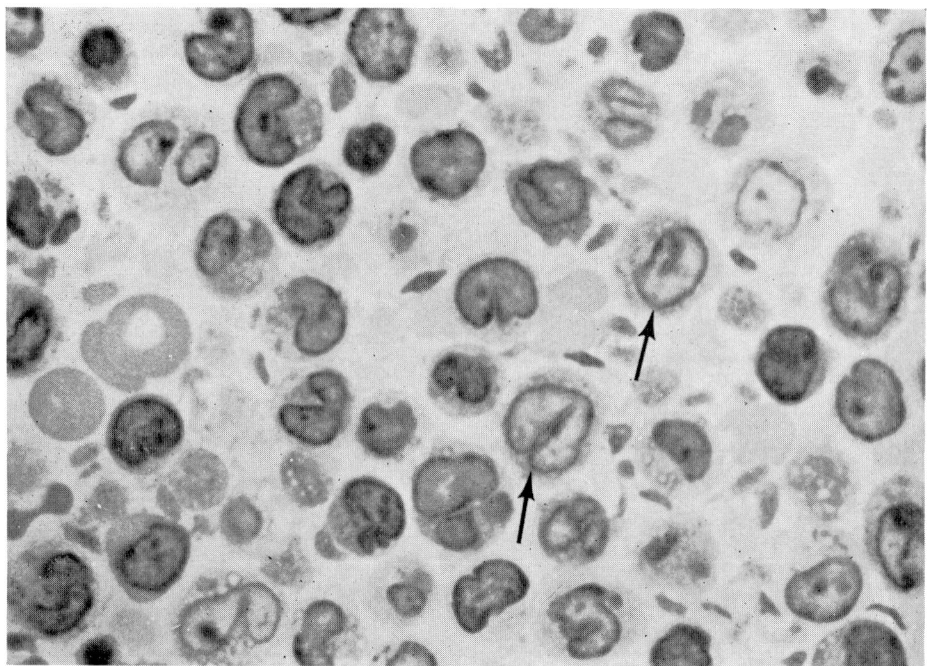

Figure 4. A one-micron-thick section of monocytes from the peripheral blood of a patient with monocytosis. The monocytes (arrows) have a slightly irregular cytoplasmic surface. Cytoplasmic granules are not seen. The nuclei have a horseshoe shape, and some contain a small to moderate amount of clumped chromatin. Nucleoli are small and inconspicuous and are seen in only a few cells.

electron microscopic appearance of the normal monocyte has been described by a number of investigators. (17,19,41,92,128,137,155,282) The ultrastructure of a typical monocyte is illustrated in Figures 5 to 7.

Electron microscopically, monocytes often have an irregular surface composed of broad-based cytoplasmic projections which may contain ribosomes, but other cytoplasmic organelles are usually lacking. Small pinocytotic vesicles as well as larger vacuoles are often seen near the cell surface. The nucleus is frequently indented and horseshoe shaped, and a nucleolus is seen in many of the cells. The chromatin shows considerable clumping around the periphery of the nucleus and patchy clumping in the central parts. Intracytoplasmic bundles of microfibrils (4,72,92,128,282) are present around the nucleus in many cells (Figs. 5–7). The area occupied by the fibrils is usually devoid of organelles. Golgi complexes and centrioles are seen, especially within the region of the nuclear concavity. Mitochondria are randomly scattered throughout the cytoplasm. A small to moderate

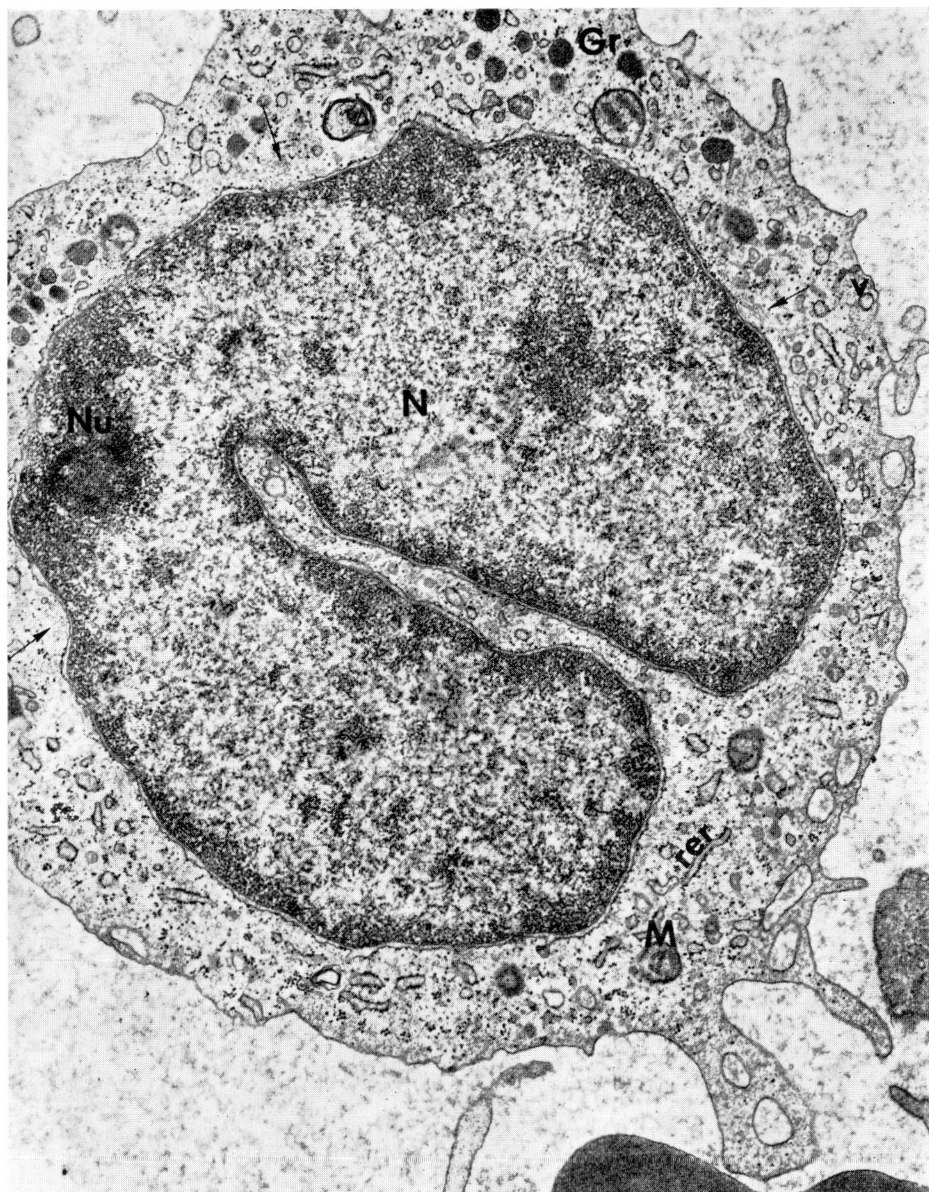

Figure 5. Electron micrograph of a normal monocyte from the peripheral blood. The indented, bean-shaped nucleus (N) contains a moderate amount of aggregated chromatin predominantly along the nuclear membrane. A small nucleolus (Nu) is present. The cell surface is irregular with plump projections of cytoplasm which contain scattered ribosomes but are devoid of other organelles. Randomly scattered small granules (Gr) which are round, oval or elongated, mitochondria (M), short segments of rough endoplasmic reticulum (rer), and micropinocytotic vesicles (v) are present in the cytoplasm. Small bundles of microfilaments (arrows) which have been cut tangentially or horizontally are seen in focal areas in the cytoplasm along the nucleus.

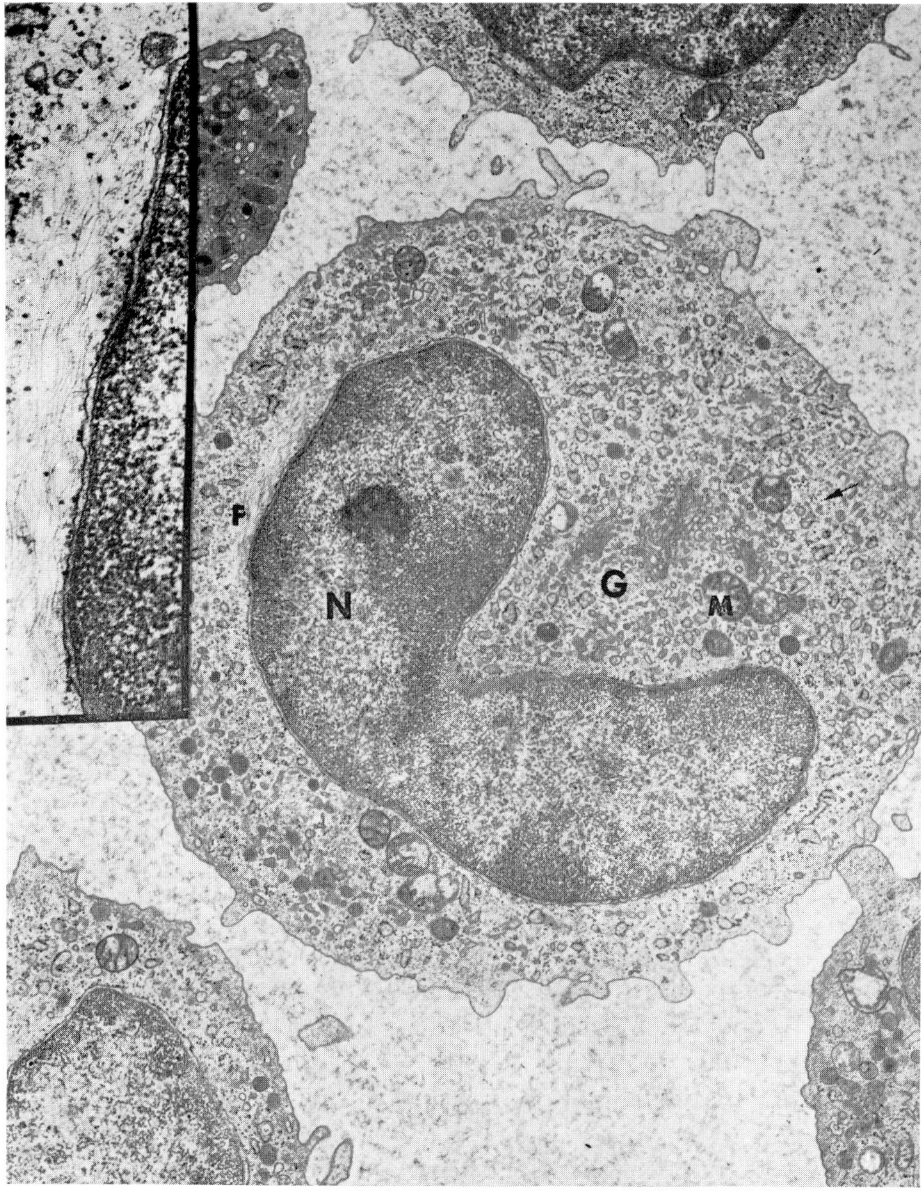

Figure 6. Monocyte from peripheral blood. The surface of the cell has multiple short, stubby projections of cytoplasm devoid of organelles. The nucleus (N) is bean-shaped, and there is a moderate amount of clumping of chromatin especially along the nuclear membrane and extending into deeper parts of the nucleus. The nucleolus is prominent. Golgi complexes (G) and many Golgi vesicles are seen in the cytoplasm of the nuclear concavity. Randomly scattered through the cytoplasm are mitochondria (M), small, round, oval and elongated moderately electron-dense granules, short segments of rough endoplasmic reticulum, free ribosomes (arrows), and pinocytotic vesicles. Bundles of microfilaments (F) course in the perinuclear part of the cytoplasm parallel to the nuclear membrane. *Inset.* Higher magnification showing perinuclear cytoplasm with bundles of microfilaments. Occasional ribosomes are present between the filaments.

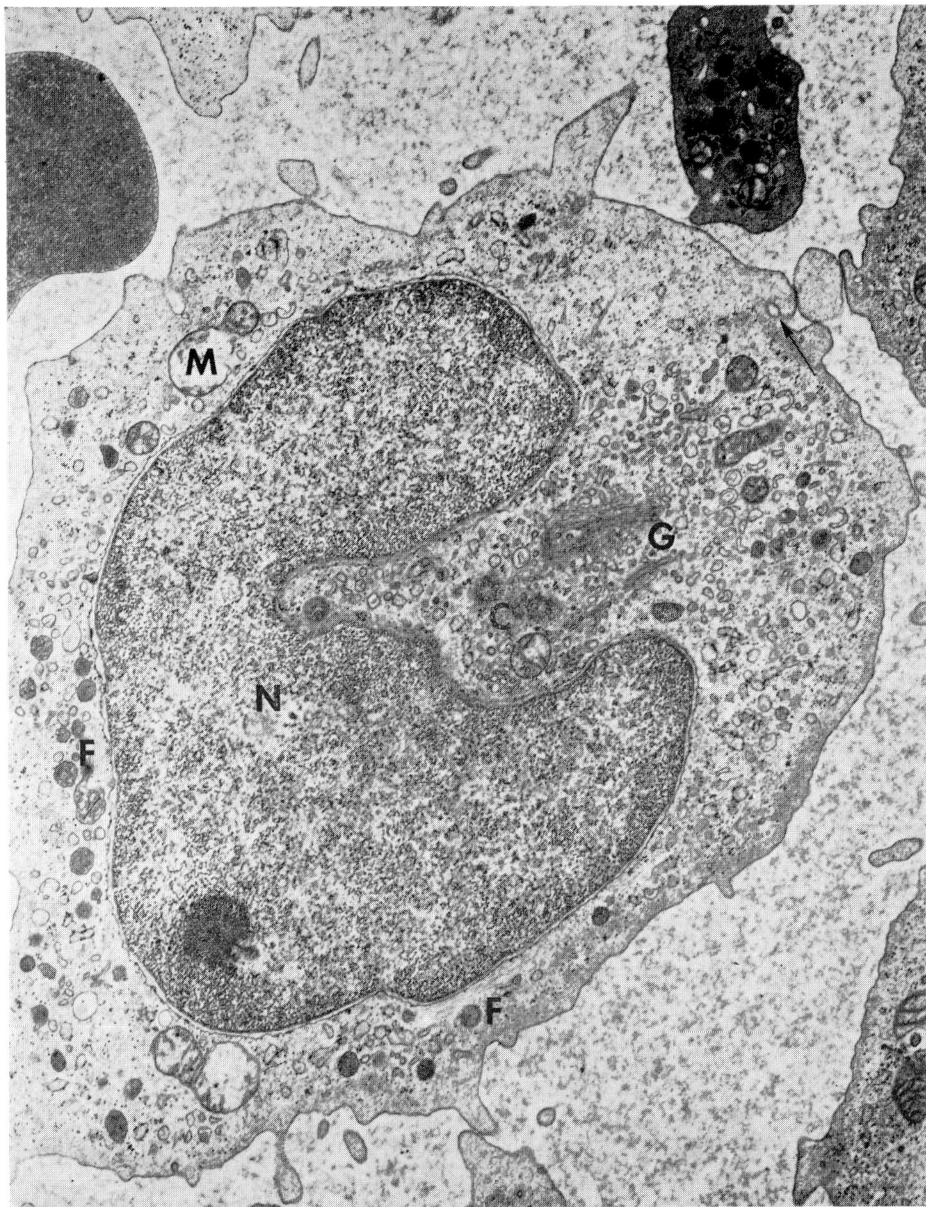

Figure 7. Monocyte from peripheral blood. The surface of the cell has a number of short, stubby projections which are devoid of cytoplasmic organelles. The nucleus (N) is indented and bean shaped and has clumping of chromatin along the nuclear membrane. A prominent small nucleolus is present. Within the cytoplasm of the nuclear concavity, there are a pair of centrioles (C), and a Golgi complex (G) with many smooth-surfaced vesicles. Mitochondria (M) are scattered randomly throughout the cytoplasm as are short segments of rough endoplasmic reticulum, free ribosomes, smooth membranes, vesicles, pinocytotic vesicles (arrow) and round, oval or elongated granules of moderate electron-density. In several areas of the cytoplasm adjacent to the nucleus, bundles of microfilaments (F) course parallel to the nuclear membrane.

number of electron-dense, round, oval or elongated granules are seen in the cytoplasm. Also present in the cytoplasm are short segments of rough endoplasmic reticulum with slightly dilated cisternae, polyribosomes and monoribosomes.

Hemohistioblast, Hemohistiocytes and Reticulum Cells

Hemohistioblasts, hemohistiocytes and reticulum cells are believed to be related both structurally and functionally to the monocytes. Forms which appear to be transitional between these cell types are seen frequently in the monocytic leukemias (Chapter III).

A normal hemohistioblast from the bone marrow as described by Ferrata (93,94) is illustrated in Figure 8a. It shows a coarsely fenes-

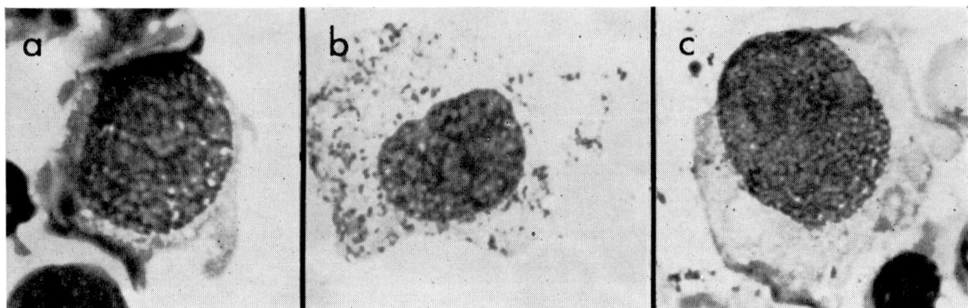

Figure 8. (a) normal hemohistioblast, (b) normal hemohistiocyte, (c) normal reticulum cell.

trated chromatin network which stains magenta in Wright's stain, and basophilic, rough-appearing cytoplasm. Several light-blue staining nucleoli may be present. Ferrata believed that the hemohistioblast could function as a "stem cell."

The normal hemohistiocyte also described by Ferrata and illustrated in Figure 8b shows a nucleus similar to that seen in the hemohistioblast, but the cytoplasm is more abundant, stains slightly eosinophilic with Wright's stain, and contains numerous azurophil granules as well as bluish-staining fibrillar structures.

The reticulum cell (Fig. 8c) shows an oval nucleus with chromatin strands which are finer and closer together than those in the hemohistiocyte or hemohistioblast. In addition, the cytoplasm is abundant and stains lightly basophilic with Wright's or Giemsa stain.

Biochemistry

Utilizing monocytes and mononuclear phagocytes obtained from rabbit peritoneal exudates, Bennett and Cohen (12) performed a series of studies relating to the content of the granules of monocytes. Their studies demonstrated that the monocyte granules, presumably lysosomes, contain a number of enzymes, such as cytochrome oxidase, acid phosphatase, aryl sulfatase, DPN hydrolase, acid DNA-ase, acid RNA-ase, beta-galactosidase, beta-glucoronidase, beta-N-acetyl-glycosamidase, cathepsin D, lipase and lysozyme.

Cytochemistry

A number of cytochemical reactions have been described as characteristic of the monocyte. (6,143,144,146,254,257,307) Some of these reactions are illustrated in Plate 3. The normal monocyte stained supravitally with neutral red and Janus green (243) appears in Plate 3a. Characteristically it is a large cell with vesicular, pale, indented nucleus and pale cytoplasm with multiple pseudopodia and ruffled borders. Multiple orange-colored vacuoles representing accumulations of neutral red are arranged in a rosette pattern. Surrounding these vacuoles are numerous rod-shaped mitochondria which have been stained with Janus green.

Plate 3b depicts the peroxidase reaction (6,35,144,291) carried out on a normal monocyte. Most normal monocytes contain less peroxidase positive material than do granulocytes. However, since monocytes, granulocytic precursors and polymorphonuclear leukocytes are peroxidase positive, they cannot be definitely distinguished from one another by means of the peroxidase reaction. Other cytochemical reactions, such as the nonspecific esterase reactions, are helpful in differentiating monocytes from granulocytic cells. Monocytes are known to exhibit nonspecific esterase activity in their cytoplasm (143, 144,145,146,235,254,255,256) when alpha-naphthyl acetate or napthol-AS-acetate is used as substrate (Plate 3c). In contrast, granulocytes contain little or no esterase-positive material with these substrates. In distinction to other bone marrow and blood cells, naphthol-AS-esterase activity is almost completely inhibited in the monocyte by sodium fluoride. Therefore the addition of sodium fluoride to the incubation media further enhances specificity of this enzyme for the monocyte. (255,257)

The esterase reaction using naphthol-AS-D chloroacetate as substrate is usually negative, although at times a small amount of reactivity is present in monocytes, while in granulocytic cells a strong reaction is seen. Sudan black stains may be positive or negative in monocytes and periodic-acid-Schiff (PAS) stains are generally negative, although an occasional monocyte shows coarsely positive granules in the cytoplasm. (257) Alkaline phosphatase activity in monocytes is negative. (257)

Schmalzl and Braunsteiner (257) have reviewed the cytochemistry of monocytes in detail. They noted that there was no metachromatic staining in monocytes using toluidine blue. Using the sulfide-silver technique, a positive iron reaction is found in monocytes, but zinc and copper have not been demonstrated. In the glycolytic pathway, glucose-6 phosphate and 6-phospho-gluconate dehydrogenase enzyme activity is intermediate between neutrophils (very active) and lymphocytes (very weak).

Choline dehydrogenase is active in certain monocytes when phenazine methosulfate is used as a mediator. Succinate, NAS-linked isocitrate and NAS-linked malate dehydrogenase show strong activities in monocytes. The authors conclude that monocytes show a less active pentose cycle but a considerably more active tricarboxylic acid cycle and a more active Embden-Meyerhof pathway than neutrophils. Monocytes, in particular, have a very high glucose requirement.

Acid phosphatase activity is high in monocytes and is localized in small granules and in some of the Golgi vesicles. Monocytes also possess beta-glucuronidase activity, weak sulfatase activity and especially high activity of acetylglucosaminidase. Lipase and phosphorylase activities are weak in monocytes, and uridine diphosphoglucose-glycogen transglycosylase activity is not detectable cytochemically in monocytes. At pH 7.15, monocytes demonstrate strong fibrinolytic activity and strong plasminogen-like activity.

Using cytochemical techniques in which peroxidase, naphthol-AS esterase, and naphthol AS-D chloracetate esterase activities were determined in the same cell, Leder (144) found that intermediate forms existed between the progranulocyte and the monocyte, and theorized that the progranulocyte was the precursor of the monocyte. These views are in accordance with those of Naegeli. (197) Rohr, (230) Heckner (122) and Schmalzl and Braunsteiner (255) were of the same opinion.

Associations between these cytochemical properties of monocytes and their function are of particular interest. The increased activity of tricarboxylic acid cycle and Embden-Meyerhof pathways along with high acetylglucosaminidase and nonspecific esterase activity reflect the capacity of the monocyte to utilize these energy pathways and enzymatic reactions in the process of phagocytosis and digestion of various types of intracellular substances. (12,50,52)

Physiology

Monocyte Locomotion

Maximow (166) and Lewis and Lewis (151) were among the first to describe the movement of mononuclear cells, presumably both lymphocytes and monocytes, in tissue cultures. Lewis and Lewis (151) noted that pseudopods appeared to thrust out of the cytoplasm of the monocyte and then retract. This sluggish ameboid-type movement did not appear to have direction as in the polymorphonuclear leukocyte but appeared random. These authors also noted the deformability of the nucleus as the cell moved. Recent time-lapse pictures by Bessis, (15) Cohn et al. (51,52,53,54) and Tompkins (284) illustrate similar phenomena.

Normal living monocytes as viewed under the phase contrast microscope are shown in Figure 9. The normal living monocyte moves

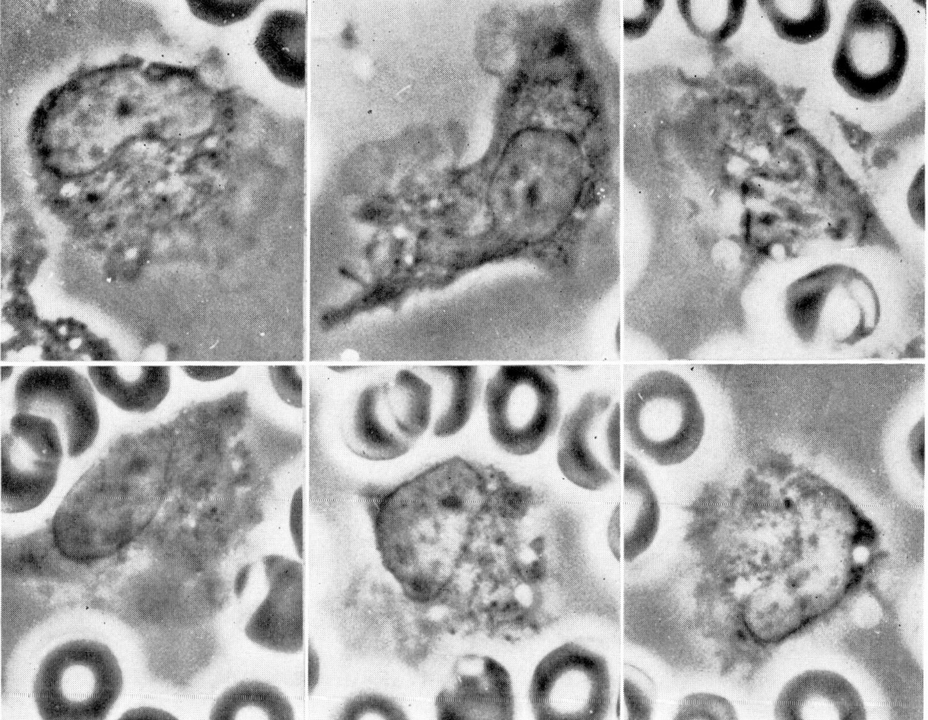

Figure 9. Phase contrast photomicrographs of living monocytes in a wet mount of normal human capillary peripheral blood. The nuclei are pale and vesicular with a dark-staining nucleolus and occasional condensations of chromatin around the nuclear membrane. The nucleus is often elongated and frequently has one or more indentations. The cytoplasm is abundant, with numerous dark-appearing, granular structures, many of which represent mitochondria. Occasionally vacuoles are seen within the cytoplasm of some of these monocytes. There are undulating cytoplasmic borders at the advancing end of the cell. The cells move sluggishly and randomly, and the pseudopodia appear to be continuously thrust out and retracted.

slowly, thrusting out and then retracting multiple pseudopodia of various sizes, some of which appear flagellar. A ruffled border of clear ectoplasm at the advancing edge of the cell is usually present. Numerous mitochondria appearing as dark punctate structures can be seen in the cytoplasm. The nucleus appears pale and vesicular and almost invariably has one or two indentations. Several aggregates of chromatin and occasionally a nucleolus can be seen. The nucleus is easily deformed as the cell moves, and multiple cytoplasmic vacuoles are frequently observed. Other investigators (52,53,54,83) have demonstrated that many of these vacuoles are actually micropinocytotic vesicles. The cell does not appear to move in a rapid unidirectional manner as do polymorphonuclear leukocytes but rather thrusts out multiple pseudopodia, moving slowly in a confined area.

Monocyte Kinetics

Studies relating to the turnover rate of monocytes have been described by Van Furth and Cohn. (290)   Utilizing radioisotopic techniques with tritium-labelled thymidine, these investigators showed that monocytes obtained from the peripheral blood were incapable of multiplication. However, they found that monocytes from bone marrow could divide and were probably the source of peripheral blood monocytes. They calculated the half-life of monocytes to be twenty-two hours. Whitelow (300) determined that the monocyte turnover rate in rats was 3.6×10^6 cells per day.

Volkman (295) observed that rat peritoneal macrophages were derived from blood monocytes. Volkman and Gowans (294) located the precursor cells of peripheral blood monocytes and tissue macrophages in the bone marrow. Their isotopic studies also indicated that the lymphocyte was not a precursor of the monocyte, a concept contrary to the view held by Bloom. (27)

Tompkins (285) observed that injection of adrenal cortical extract could cause a decrease in the number of circulating monocytes. Yoshida et al. (309) found a similar decrease in blood monocyte levels after injection of intravenous antigen into animals. Monocytosis ensued after the initial monocytopenia.

Monocyte-Macrophage Transformations

Although a number of investigators, (45,220,248) notably Maximow (166,167,168) and Lewis and Lewis (151) described the development of monocytes into macrophages using tissue cultures, one of the first *in vivo* studies demonstrating the development of macrophages from peripheral blood monocytes was that of Ebert and

Florey. (82)   Using rabbit ear chambers, they noted the diapedesis of monocytes through capillaries and the eventual transformation of monocytes into macrophages capable of ingesting vital dyes. Petrakis et al. (213) also traced the development of monocytes into phagocytes. Sutton and Weiss (280) in tissue culture studies noted that chicken monocytes transformed into macrophages, epitheloid cells and giant cells.

Phagocytosis

Metchnikoff (186) was one of the first investigators to study phagocytosis by mononuclear cells. This phenomenon has been studied by others, primarily in tissue culture systems. In 1922 Simpson (273) injected colloidal dyes intravenously into rabbits and noted the appearance of typical macrophages in the peripheral blood. Eliot (87) in 1926 observed that phagocytes of various organs in the rabbit appeared to be derived from circulating mononuclear cells, presumably monocytes. An early account of phagocytosis of erythrocytes and leukocytes by mononuclear cells in the peripheral blood of human subjects was given by Van Nuys (292) in 1907 in a paper entitled *An Extraordinary Blood*. Van Nuys illustrated large mononuclear phagocytes from the peripheral blood of a patient with aortic valvular disease and fever, probably symptoms of bacterial endocarditis. An additional early report by Rowley (239) in 1908 described "A fatal anemia with enormous numbers of circulating phagocytes." Rowley noted active phagocytosis of both erythrocytes and polymorphonuclear leukocytes by "large lymphocytes." Photomicrographs of these "large lymphocytes" strongly suggest that they are monocytes.

Some of the early clinical studies of phagocytosis by mononuclear cells were those of Schilling in 1919 who described mononuclear phagocytes in the peripheral blood of patients with bacterial endocarditis. (249)   The plate from his original paper illustrating these phagocytes is reproduced in Figure 10. Phagocytosis by mononuclear cells in subacute bacterial endocarditis was also described by Pepper (211) who stated that monocytosis occurred in subacute bacterial endocarditis (SBE), and that gradations between macrophages and monocytes were seen in the peripheral blood. Hurxthal (130) saw similar "macrophages" in this condition and noted erythrophagocytosis. Ottander (207) also noted "endothelial phagocytes" in the peripheral blood of patients with SBE. Daland et al. (63) and Cole (55) found that histiocytes could be demonstrated in the first drop of capillary peripheral blood obtained from the earlobe of patients with subacute bacterial endocarditis. Hill and Bayrd (127) determined that

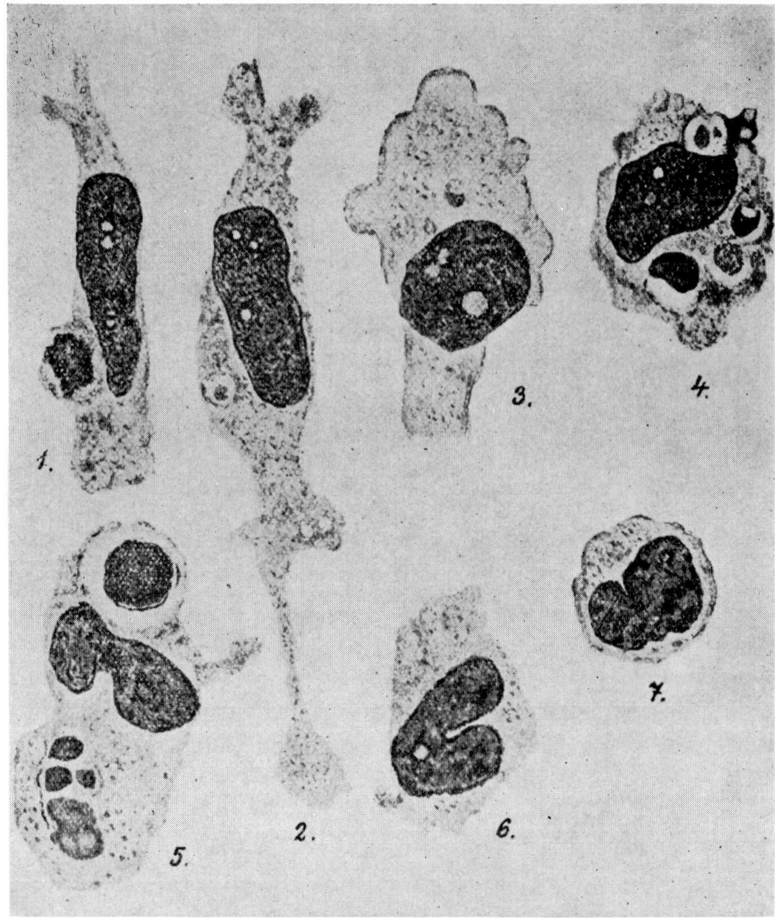

Figure 10. From Schilling (1919). Mononuclear phagocytes from a case of "endo-carditis lenta." Erythrophagocytosis is evident. (Reprinted with permission of Julius Springer Verlag.)

phagocytic reticuloendothelial cells appeared in greater numbers in patients with subacute bacterial endocarditis when their blood cultures were sterile.

Cohn et al. (51,52,53,54) detected changes in the metabolism of monocytes during their "transformation" into phagocytes. Their studies demonstrated that the "conversion" of monocytes into macrophages was accompanied by an increase in the number of lysosome-like cytoplasmic organelles. In addition, there was an increase in the activity of cytochrome oxidase, acid phosphatase, aryl sulfatase and BPN hydrolase. Glucose utilization, lactic acid and uptake of both bacteria and colloidal gold were also increased during this transformation.

In their study of phagocytosis by human monocytes, Cline and

CHAPTER IV

THE MONOCYTIC LEUKEMIAS

MORPHOLOGICALLY, there are a number of detailed features of the monocyte nucleus and cytoplasm which are seen frequently in monocytes in the monocytic leukemias. These features are rarely observed in the benign and "reactive" monocytes described in Chapter III, but rather appear to be characteristic of neoplastic monocytes. These features include large and sometimes multiple nucleoli, specific neutrophil or eosinophil granules, multiple nuclear lobulations, hemo-histiocytic-type nuclear chromatin, cytoplasmic tail, multiple pseudopodia devoid of granules and aggregates of granules in a perinuclear distribution. These characteristics are illustrated in Figure 12. They may be observed alone, or more frequently, in combination with other neoplastic morphological characteristics in any one particular neoplastic monocyte.

Cytochemical characteristics of neoplastic monocytes were studied by Hayhoe (119,120,121) and by Schmalzl and Braunsteiner. (257) Like normal monocytes, leukemic monocytes in monocytic leukemias showed high sodium fluoride-sensitive-napthol-AS esterase activity. Sudan Black B-positive lipids, peroxidase and naphthol-AS-D chloracetate esterase were weakly reactive in these leukemic cells. In addition, activity of naphthyl-amidase, alpha-napthyl-acetate esterase, NAD-H diaphorase, and isocitric and malic dehydrogenase could be demonstrated in leukemic monocytes.

Leukemic monocytes and blasts from patients with acute myelomonocytic and histiomonocytic leukemias have been shown to contain abundant amounts of lysozyme (muramidase) by immunofluorescent and immunochemical techniques (5,256,278) and by a newly developed staining technique for the direct demonstration of lysozyme in these cells. (261) The enzyme is thought to be localized in lysosomes (206,257) of these monocytes. Presumably the monocytes are the major source of the elevated urinary lysozyme levels in many patients with acute monocytic leukemia. (206)

Bodel and Atkins (31) determined that monocytes obtained from patients with agranulocytosis and with acute monocytic leukemia liberated pyrogen *in vitro* after incubation with heat-killed *staphylococcus aureus.*

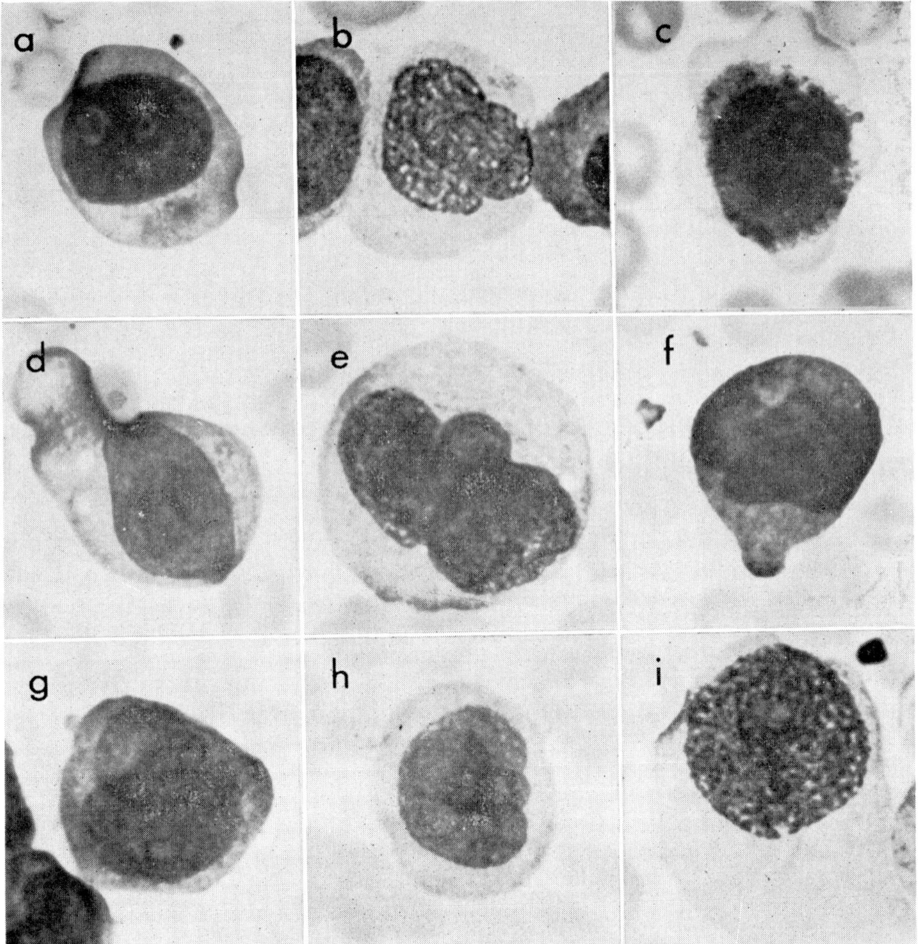

Figure 12. A variety of neoplastic monocytes obtained from patients with myelomonocytic leukemia and histiomonocytic leukemia.

(a) A "myleomonoblast." The nuclear chromatin is diffuse, and several prominent nucleoli are seen. The cytoplasm is opaque and sparsely granular.

(b) A hemohistioblast with monocytoid nucleus.

(c) A neoplastic monocyte with prominent, clear ectoplasmic pseudopodia and nonspecific granules which appear aggregated in a perinuclear distribution.

(d) A histiomonoblast. A prominent cytoplasmic tail can be seen.

(e) A bizarre-appearing, giant monocytoid cell from a patient with reticulum cell sarcoma leukemia. The nucleus is unusually large and multilobulated with prominent aggregates of chromatin.

(f) A "myelomonocyte" with prominent nuclear infoldings and lobulations. A cytoplasmic tail is seen as well as abundant neutrophilic-type cytoplasmic granules, giving this cell features of both monocytes and granulocytes.

(g) A "myelomonoblast" with unusual ballooning of the nucleus and a prominent nucleolus.

(h) A histiomonocyte with multilobulated nucleus containing delicate chromatin strands.

(i) A histiomonocyte with nucleus resembling that of a hemohistioblast. A prominent nucleolus is seen.

Lymphosarcoma Cells, Sézary Cells and Histiocytoid Lymphocytes

There are a number of cells which have certain features of neoplastic monocytes but which are not actually monocytes. Several of these cells are illustrated in Figure 13. Figure 13a shows a typical

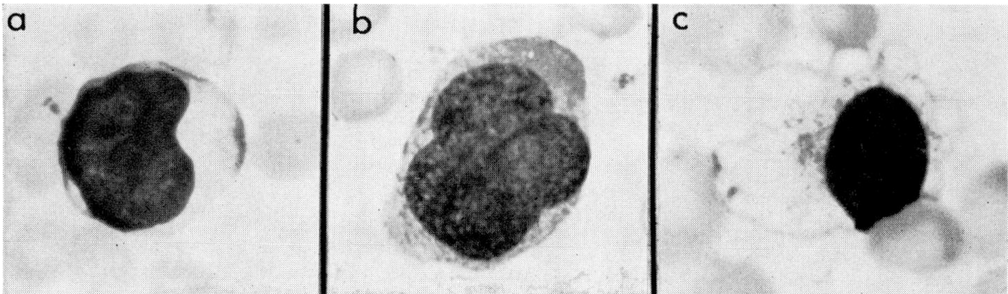

Figure 13. (a) A so-called "lymphosarcoma cell" from a patient with lymphosarcoma cell leukemia. The nucleus shows a prominent indentation and diffuse chromatin in some areas, and sponge-like chromatin in others. A large nucleolus is present. The cytoplasm is deeply basophilic and contains multiple vacuoles.

(b) A monocytoid cell from a patient with the Sézary syndrome. The nucleus shows multiple lobulations and infoldings. The chromatin strands appear coarse with occasional blocklike aggregates. The cytoplasm is opaque and granular. PAS-positive material may be seen in the cytoplasm of these cells.

(c) A histiocytoid lymphocyte from a patient with advanced lymphosarcoma. The nucleus is typically lymphoid, with blocklike and linear aggregates of chromatin. However, the cytoplasm shows undulations and appears voluminous like a histiocyte. Multiple pseudopodia such as are seen in neoplastic monocytes are also present. Nonspecific granules appear clustered in a perinuclear distribution.

"lymphosarcoma cell" from "lymphosarcoma cell" leukemia. (132) The nucleus has a prominent indentation, and the chromatin has a spongy reticular appearance. The cytoplasm is deeply basophilic and may contain vacuoles. Although the cell does have a large nucleus with a prominent indentation or fold, it is nevertheless not considered a monocyte but instead lies in the category of poorly differentiated lymphocytic lymphoma in a leukemic phase. (217) A bone marrow aspirate from a patient with this disorder is seen in Figure 14.

Figure 13b illustrates a large monocytoid-appearing cell from a patient with the Sézary syndrome. (270,271) This syndrome is said to be related to the "cutaneous reticuloses" such as mycosis fungoides. (36) The typical Sézary cell has a nucleus with multiple overlapping convolutions, resembling convolutions of the brain, and coarsely reticular chromatin. The cytoplasm is grayish-blue and is generally periodic-acid-Schiff (PAS) positive. Although superficially monocytoid in appearance and described by Sézary (270,271) as being histiomonocy-

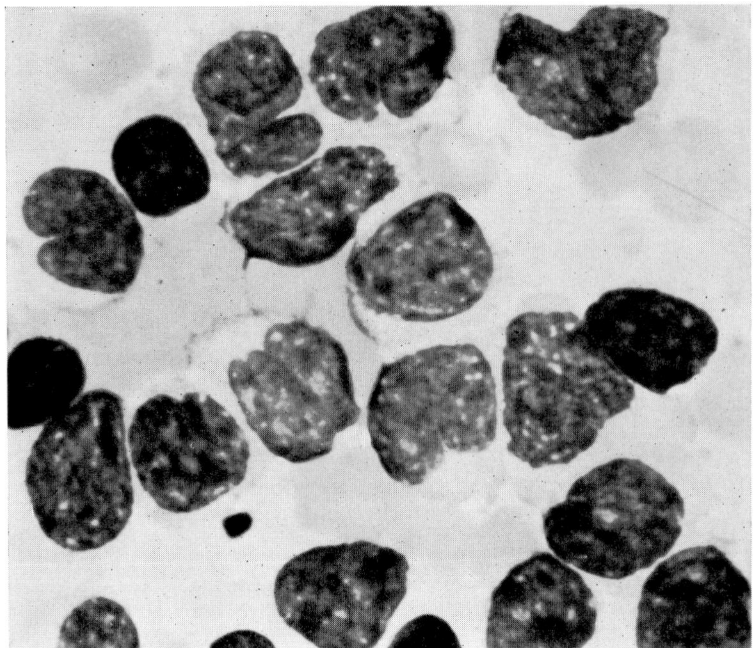

Figure 14. Lymphosarcoma cell leukemia. This photomicrograph is from the bone marrow of a patient with lymphosarcoma cell leukemia. The cells are neoplastic lymphocytes, although the indentations of their nuclei make them appear superficially monocytoid. Sharply defined aggregates of chromatin can be seen within the nuclei. The cytoplasm is opaque blue.

toid, the Sézary cell is considered by some to be an aberrant type of lymphosarcoma cell.

Figure 13c illustrates another type of cell with monocytoid features. It is a histiocytoid lymphocyte from a patient with lymphosarcoma. The nucleus is that of an intermediate lymphocyte, but the abundant foamy cytoplasm with multiple pseudopodia and clear ectoplasmic borders is characteristic of a histiocyte. Nevertheless, this cell is considered to be part of the cytological spectrum of poorly differentiated lymphocytic lymphoma (lymphosarcoma). These cells appear similar to those originally described and illustrated in 1935 by Stasney and Downey, (276) who felt that reticuloendothelial cells in patients with "subacute lymphatic leukemia" were derived from "the reticulum" and stated that certain of these cells had the cytoplasm of a reticuloendothelial cell and the nucleus of a lymphocyte.

Subacute Myelomonocytic Leukemia

In contrast to the acute forms of monocytic leukemia, the subacute form of myelomonocytic leukemia is usually a more indolent disorder.

Prolonged periods of weakness and fatigue are common prior to diagnosis. Hepatomegaly and splenomegaly are seen frequently, but lymphadenopathy is uncommon. Widespread osteolytic lesions can also occur and may be associated with severe bone pain. Soft tissue infections are especially frequent. Subacute myelomonocytic leukemia often presents as a refractory anemia, at times with leukopenia and thrombocytopenia. Generally the hemoglobin is between 7 to 10 grams percent and the white blood count is usually elevated above 10,000 mm^3. In some instances, patients may have changes diagnostic of refractory acquired sideroblastic anemia (24,62,124,293) or chronic erythemic myelosis (DiGuglielmo syndrome) several months prior to the appearance of increased numbers of monocytes in the peripheral blood. In a small number of patients, transition into acute myelomonocytic leukemia occurs from several months to as long as several years after the diagnosis of subacute myelomonocytic leukemia has been established. The majority of patients, however, succumb to either sepsis or hemorrhage or both.

Monocytosis is usually apparent in the peripheral blood even in leukopenic states, and the monocytes often exhibit many of the neoplastic features enumerated at the beginning of this chapter. This is not always the case, however, and peripheral blood monocytes in subacute myelomonocytic leukemia may appear morphologically normal. Occasionally large bizarre-appearing hypergranular platelets may be found in the peripheral blood. Progranulocytes, myelocytes and metamyelocytes are seen infrequently. Aberrant-appearing polymorphonuclear leukocytes are sometimes observed. These cells have prominent basophilic granulation in their cytoplasm and bizarre-appearing nuclear lobulations. Some may show an acquired Pelger-Huet anomaly of nuclear segmentation. (71)

The erythrocytes in the peripheral blood show considerable anisocytosis and poikilocytosis. Macrocytosis of erythrocytes is more common than in acute myelomonocytic and histiomonocytic leukemias. Large macroovalocytes and irregularly shaped, unusually large macrocytes as well as nucleated red cells are sometimes seen.

Although myeloblasts are seen in this disorder, the predominant cell has a monocytoid nucleus often with multiple lobulations, opaque lavender-gray cytoplasm and innumerable granules, many of which appear to be specific neutrophil granules as seen in Figure 12.

The leukemic cells in sections of Epon-embedded peripheral blood from patients with subacute myelomonocytic leukemia are characterized by very irregular nuclei and small granules within the cytoplasm. Evidence of erythrophagocytosis by leukemic cells is occasionally seen (Fig. 15). Ultrastructurally, most of the leukemic cells have an ir-

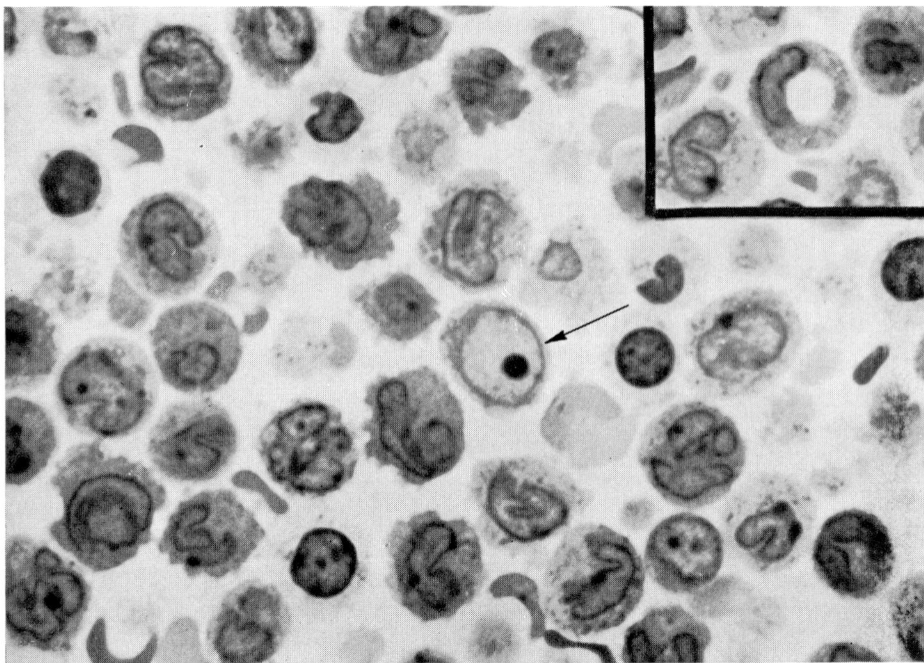

Figure 15. A one-micron-thick section of peripheral blood from a patient with subacute myelomonocytic leukemia. The leukemic cells have a smooth or irregular cytoplasmic surface and ample cytoplasm. Most of the nuclei are very irregular in shape, and nucleoli are either small or not seen at all. Some of the cells contain horseshoe-shaped nuclei. One immature cell (arrow) has a large, oval nucleus with little chromatin and a large, prominent nucleus in its center. Small granules are seen scattered within the cytoplasm of many cells. *Inset.* Erythrophagocytosis by a leukemic cell.

regular surface (Fig. 16). Many of the nuclei are irregular in shape, some are indented and others have a horseshoe shape. Aggregated chromatin is seen mostly at the periphery of the nucleus, but some is also present deeper within the nucleus. Nucleoli are generally small. Some cells have nuclear blebs (Figs. 16b, 17, 18) or nuclear fragments connected to the main part of the nucleus by a nuclear strand or bridge. The nuclear blebs or loops in some cells are large, encompassing much of the cell's cytoplasm. Nuclear blebs and bridges have been described in monocytic (102,171) and granulocytic leukemias. (16,18,21) Granules are seen in the cytoplasm of many leukemic cells (Figs. 16–19). Some of these cells which appear to belong to the granulocytic series are hypogranular and often have abnormally shaped nuclei (Fig. 16).

Typically, the bone marrows from patients with subacute myelomonocytic leukemias show panmyelosis. The association of increased proerythroblasts, megaloblastoid intermediate macronormoblasts,

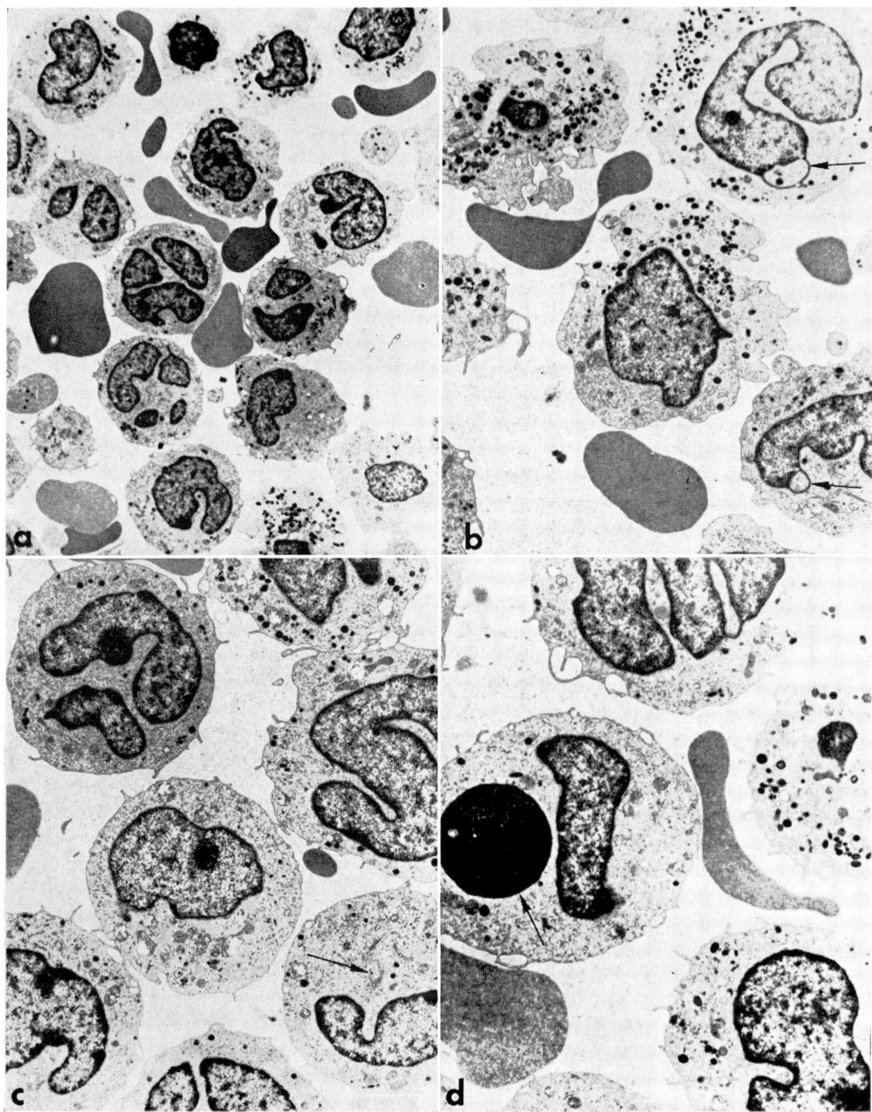

Figure 16. Peripheral blood from a patient with subacute myelomonocytic leukemia. (a) and (b) The surface indentations of the cytoplasm give the leukemic cells an irregular shape. The nuclei are either irregular, indented, or horseshoe-shaped. A moderate amount of clumping of chromatin is seen along the periphery of the nucleus but also scattered throughout the nucleus. Small nucleoli are seen in some cells. Nuclear blebs (short arrows) are evident in two cells. Some of the cells have many oval, round or elongated dense granules, most of which are concentrated in one part of the cytoplasm, while other cells have relatively few granules. (c) Leukemic cells showing irregular shapes of the nuclei. The cell in the center appears to be less mature than others and is characterized by an irregularly shaped nucleus containing a prominent nucleolus, mitochondria polarized in one part of the cytoplasm and relatively few small granules. Prominent Golgi complexes and a centriole are seen in one cell (long arrow). A moderate number of ribosomes, a few segments of rough endoplasmic reticulum and a number of vacuoles are seen in the cytoplasm. (d) One of the leukemic cells contains a phagocytized red cell in its cytoplasm.

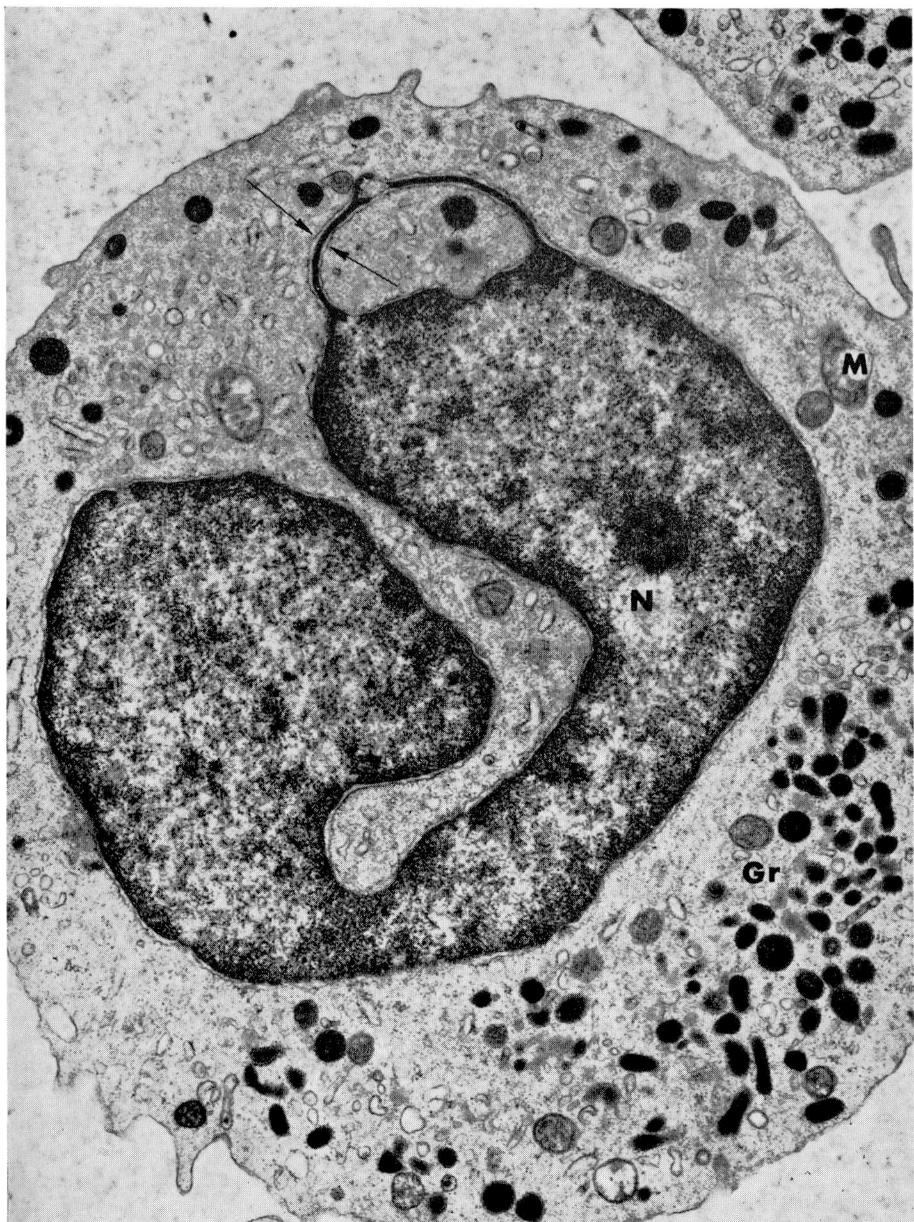

Figure 17. Higher magnification of one of the cells seen in Figure 16b. The deeply indented nucleus (N) has a moderate amount of condensed chromatin, a small nucleolus and a nuclear bleb. The nuclear membrane (arrows) surrounding the heterochromatin is clearly seen. Most of the granules (Gr), which vary in size and shape, are present in one part of the cytoplasm. Scattered ribosomes and mitochondria (M) are present.

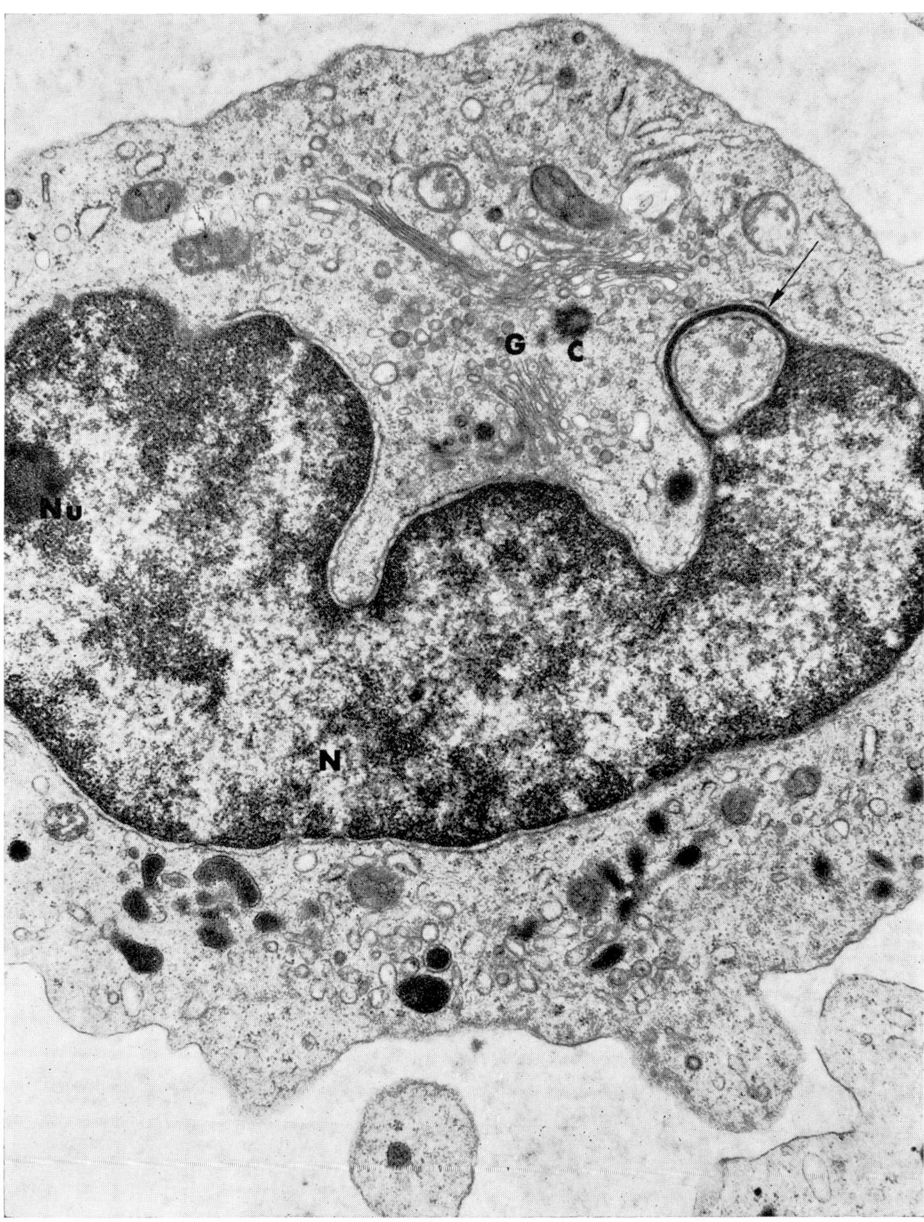

Figure 18. Higher magnification of one of the cells seen in Figure 16b. The indented nucleus (N) has a nuclear bleb (arrow). Golgi complexes (G) surround a centriole (C) in the cytoplasm of the nuclear concavity. A small number of irregularly shaped, dense granules are seen in the cytoplasm.

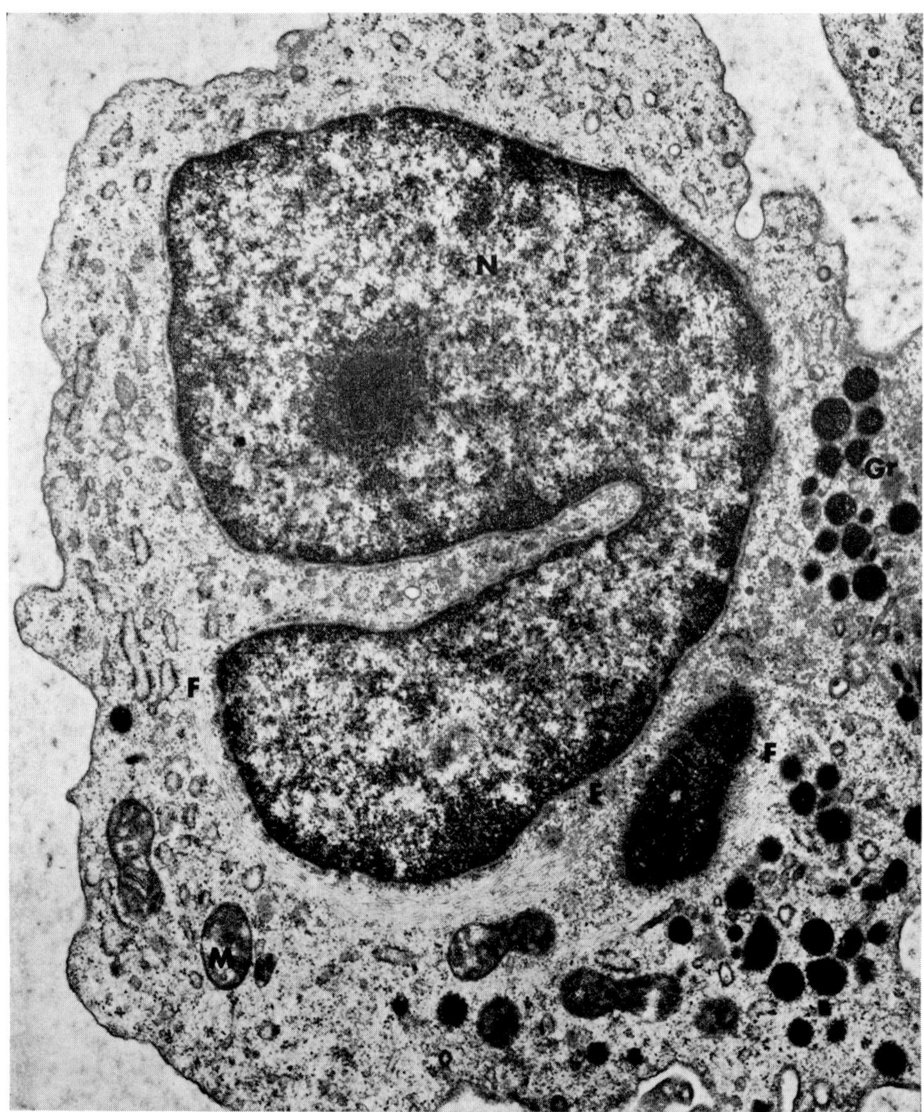

Figure 19. An irregularly shaped leukemic cell with a horseshoe-shaped nucleus (N) and a small nuclear fragment whose connection to the main nucleus is not visible. A prominent nucleolus is seen. A bundle of microfilaments (F) course around part of the nucleus in the perinuclear cytoplasm. Round and oval dense granules (Gr) are localized in one part of the cytoplasm which also contains mitochondria (M), rough endoplasmic reticulum and scattered ribosomes.

plasma cells and neoplastic monocytes is particularly common (Fig. 20). Aberrations in granulocyte precursors in subacute myelomonocytic leukemia are frequent. Granulopoiesis is generally left-shifted, with increased numbers of progranulocytes and myelocytes. The granulocyte

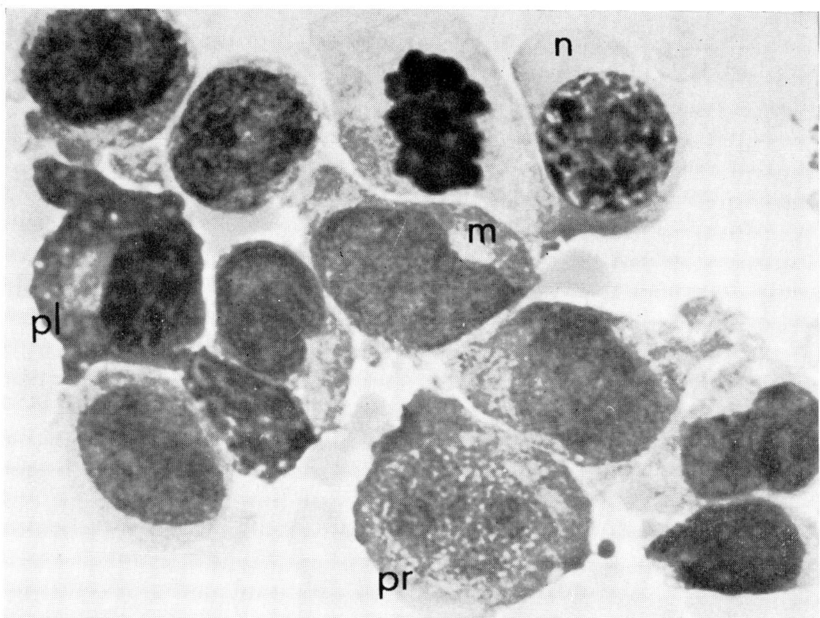

Figure 20. Subacute myelomonocytic leukemia. A combination of cells which are frequently seen in subacute myelomonocytic leukemia. Plasma cells (pl), proerythroblasts (pr), megaloblastoid intermediate macronormoblasts (n), neoplastic "myelomonocytes" (m) and mitotic figures are frequently seen together.

precursors may show a variety of changes, all of which may be considered to be neoplastic (Fig. 21). Some of the changes, illustrated in Figure 21, include extensive foldings and loopings of the nucleus of a monocyte or progranulocyte; myelocytes with monocytoid nuclei; and specific neutrophil, eosinophil or basophil granules in hemohistiocytes and hemohistioblasts. Auer rods are sometimes seen in these cells as shown in Figures 22a and 22c. Cells containing features of other cells ("basoeosinophils") are sometimes found. Large, unusual-appearing monocytoid cells which present difficulty as to their designation as monocytic or monocytoid progranulocytic cells are seen frequently (Fig. 23).

Increased numbers of hemohistiocytes, reticulum cells and hemohistioblasts are frequent, as seen in Figure 24. Many of these cells have monocytoid nuclei with elaborate nuclear foldings and indentations (Fig. 25) and often contain specific neutrophil or eosinophil myeloid granules in their cytoplasm.

Aberrations in megakarocytes are commonly associated, and a spectrum of changes is illustrated in Figure 26. Giant, bizarre megakaryocytes, small binucleate forms and megakaryocytes with mono-

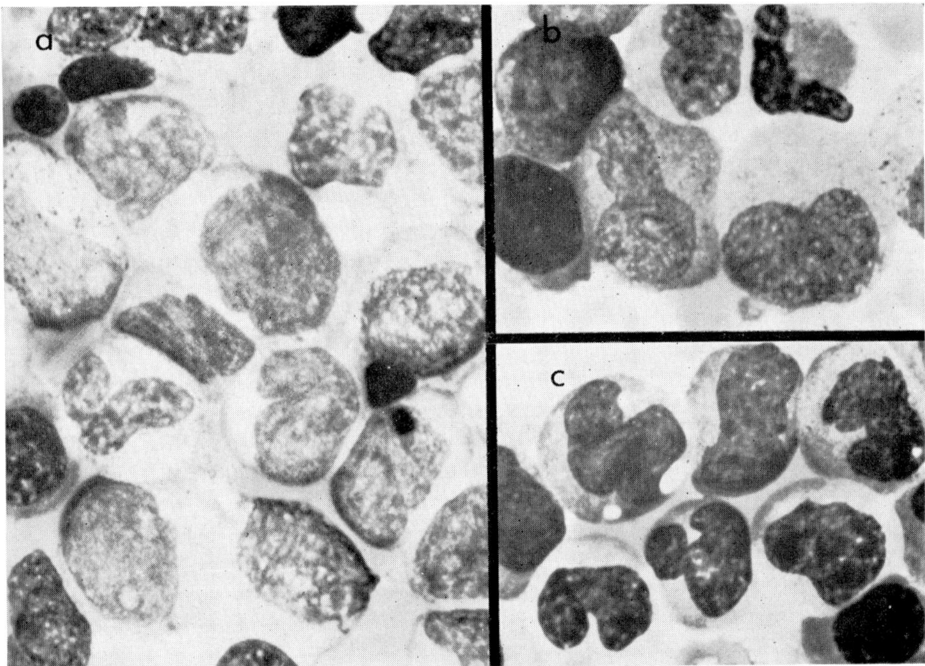

Figure 21. Aberrations in myelocytes, metamyelocytes and band forms in three patients with subacute myelomonocytic leukemia. Unusual monocytoid-type twistings and foldings of the nuclei of these cells are observed.

cytoid nuclei are seen. Megakaryocytes with coarsely reticular nuclei resembling those of hemohistiocytes or hemohistioblasts can sometimes be observed, as seen in Figure 26. It is uncertain whether or not the polymorphonuclear leukocytes and erythrocytes in the cytoplasm of some of these megakaryocytes represent phagocytosis or so-called "emperipolesis." (219)

Abnormalities in the number or morphology of erythroid precursors are especially common in subacute myelomonocytic leukemia. Hyperplasia of proerythroblasts is frequent, as seen in Figure 27A, and large multinucleate erythroid forms can be found (Fig. 27B). As illustrated in Figure 28A, the type of erythropoiesis is most often megaloblastoid, with chromatin features as described in Chapter VI. It is conceivable that these megaloblastoid cells represent the source of the unusually large and bizarre-shaped macrocytes in the peripheral blood of these patients (Fig. 28B). Multinucleate megaloblastoid intermediate macronormoblasts, giant megaloblastoid forms and late normoblasts with coarse basophilic stippling are also seen frequently (Fig. 29). Late normoblasts with aberrant mitoses are also observed.

Increased numbers of mature-appearing plasma cells are often

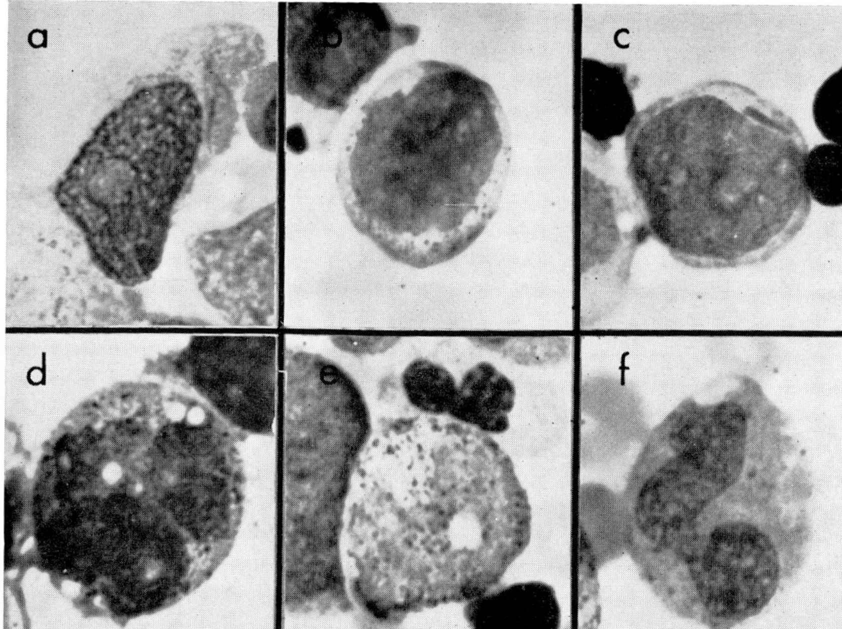

Figure 22. Granulocyte aberrations in myelomonocytic leukemias.

(a) Hemohistiocyte with prominent nucleolus and Auer rod.

(b) Blast with prominent cytoplasmic granules and clear-blue cytoplasm.

(c) Blast with prominent nucleoli and Auer rod.

(d) Monocyte with multiple nuclear lobulations resembling a cloverleaf pattern, and vacuolated cytoplasm containing specific neutrophil granules.

(e) Metamyelocyte with doughnut-shaped nucleus.

(f) Metamyelocyte with unusual twisting of the nucleus and bulbous end.

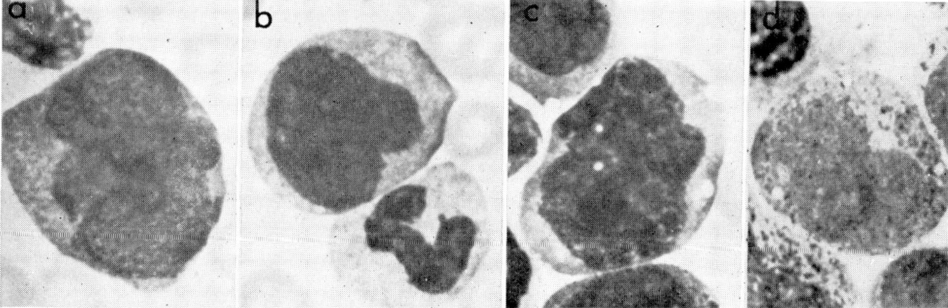

Figure 23. Unusual monocytoid cells in subacute myelomonocytic leukemia.

(a) Unusually large monocytoid cell with prominent nucleoli and multiple nuclear lobulations.

(b) Monocytoid cell with large, blocklike aggregates of nuclear chromatin and agranular cytoplasm.

(c) Monocytoid cell with extensively aggregated nuclear chromatin and multilobulation of the nucleus.

(d) Cell with convoluted monocytoid nucleus and cytoplasm containing specific neutrophil granules ("monocytoid progranulocyte").

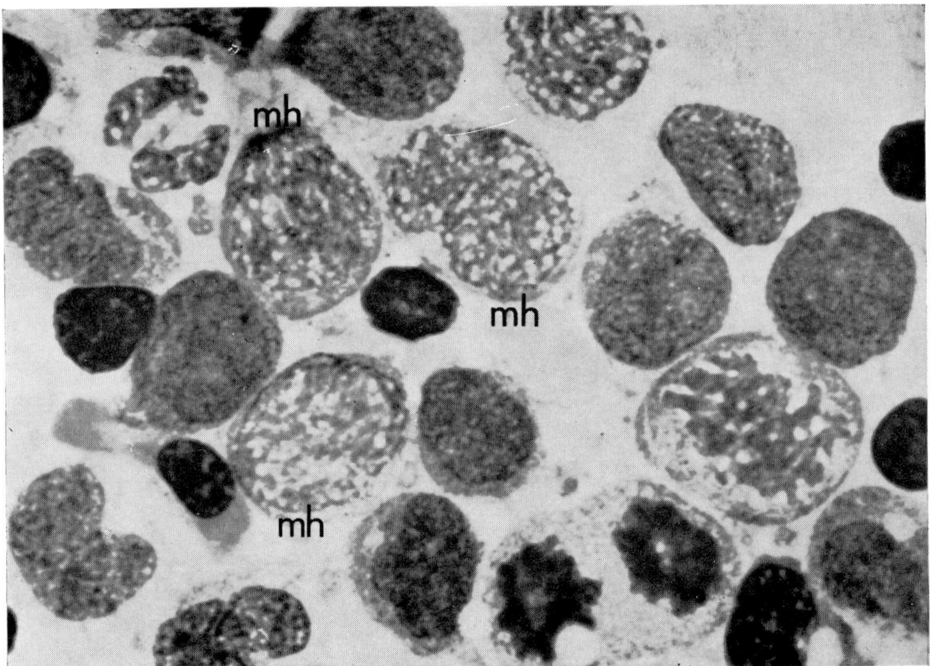

Figure 24. Hemohistiocytes and hemohistioblasts with monocytoid nuclei (mh) and neoplastic monocytes are seen. Several mitotic figures appear at the lower right.

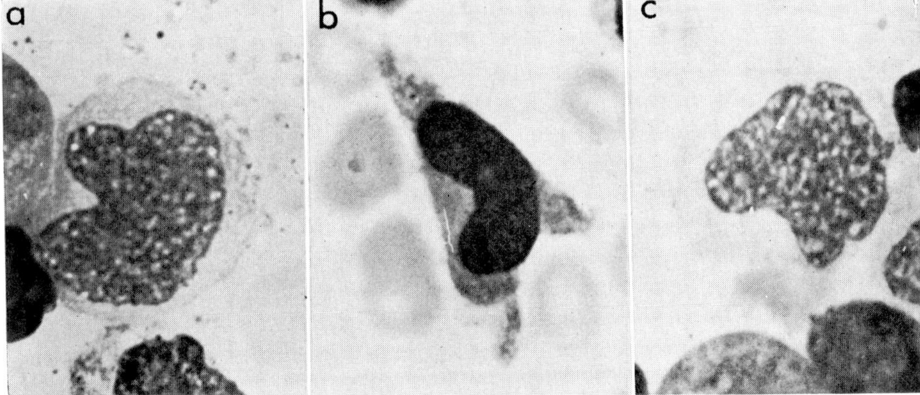

Figure 25. Hemohistiocytic abnormalities in monocytic leukemias. These three photomicrographs show monocytoid changes in hemohistioblasts, reticulum cells and hemohistiocytes in subacute myelomonocytic leukemia. Multiple indentations and infoldings of the nuclei can be seen.

seen in subacute myelomonocytic leukemia (Fig. 30). At times, the cytoplasm of these plasma cells may contain numerous large vacuoles.

The variability in the clinical course of patients with myelomonocytic leukemia has been commented upon by various investigators, particularly Sinn and Dick, (275) and more recently Saarni and Linman, (242) Linman (152) and Bennett. (11) In a group of patients with the diagnosis of subacute myelomonocytic leukemia followed for varying periods of time at the Simpson Memorial Institute of the University of Michigan, survival ranged from six months to as long as forty-four months after diagnosis. Patients in this series showed infrequent evolution into an acute myelomonocytic or myeloblastic type of leukemia. The majority of patients succumbed to either hemorrhage or sepsis or both.

Because of this variability in the clincial course of myelomonocytic leukemias, Saarni and Linman (242) and Linman (152) have preferred to designate all types of myelomonocytic leukemia, acute and presumably subacute, as simply myelomonocytic leukemia. They believe that the disorder represents a broad spectrum of clinical manifestations and do not attempt to further classify myelomonocytic leukemia on the basis of morphological abnormalities (percentage of blast forms, etc.) or aggressiveness of clinical behavior.

Our impression is that although subacute myelomonocytic leukemia may fit within the broad framework of myelomonocytic leukemias in general, its morphological and clinical features are distinctive enough to justify its designation as an entity separate from the more aggressive acute myelomonocytic leukemia.

Chronic Monocytic Leukemia

Certain cases of monocytic leukemia called by various terms including "chronic monocytic leukemia" (9,215,241) and "chronic erythromonocytic leukemia" (37) also appear to be similar to what we consider to be subacute myelomonocytic leukemia. In 1940 Wintrobe and Mitchell (304) included a patient with hepatomegaly, indurated skin lesions and monocytosis in a review of atypical manifestations of leukemia. They concluded that "the case seems to be typical of monocytic leukemia, although less acute than is usually seen."

In 1951 Beattie et al. (9) described what they called "chronic monocytic leukemia" in an individual who had refractory anemia and monocytosis with a particularly indolent clinical course. In 1956 Sinn and Dick (275) described a series of cases characterized by refractory, often macrocytic, anemia and monocytosis and a similar protracted course. The cases described by Wintrobe and Mitchell,

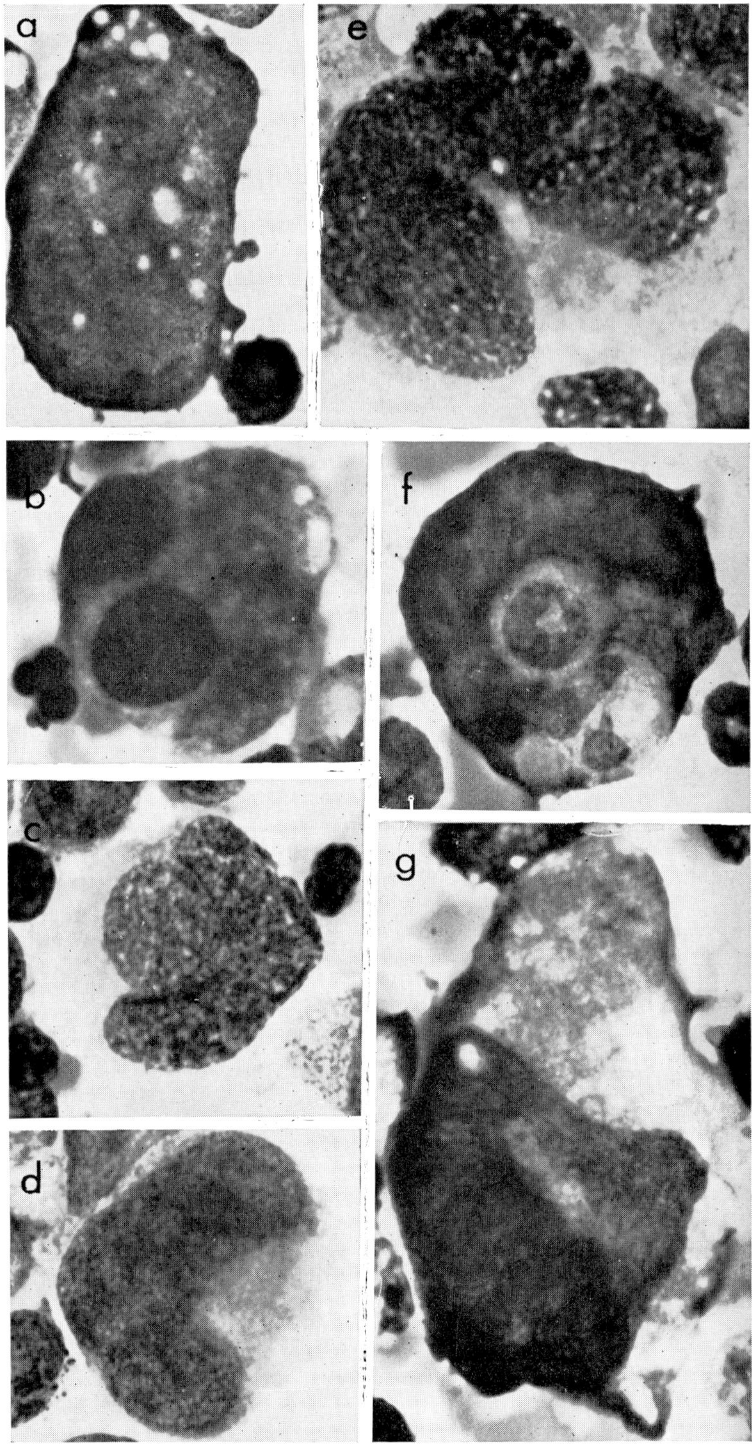

Figure 26. Megakaryocytic abnormalities in myelomonocytic leukemias.

(a) A megakaryocyte from a patient with acute myelomonocytic leukemia. The nucleus is unusually large with diffuse chromatin. The cytoplasm contains several vacuoles, and abortive platelet formation is seen along one of the cell margins.

(b) A megakaryocyte from a patient with subacute myelomonocytic leukemia. Two small, disconnected lobes are seen. The cytoplasm shows normal granulation, but it appears unusually clumped.

(c) A megakaryocyte from a patient with acute myelomonocytic leukemia. The nuclear lobes appear multiple and compacted into one end of the cell. The chromatin appears somewhat fenestrated with only occasional aggregates.

(d) A megakaryocyte from a patient with subacute myelomonocytic leukemia. The nucleus contains several infoldings, and the cytoplasm is hypogranular.

(e) A megakaryocyte from a patient with subacute myelomonocytic leukemia. The nuclear chromatin is unusually coarse, resembling that seen in a hemohistiocyte. Several lobulations are seen. The cytoplasm is voluminous and poorly granular.

(f) A megakaryocyte from a patient with acute histiomonocytic leukemia, showing phagocytosis (? emperipolesis) of polymorphonuclear leukocytes by a megakaryocyte.

(g) An unusually large megakaryocyte from a patient with acute histiomonocytic leukemia. The nucleus shows diffuse strands of chromatin, and the lobes appear to be compressed into one end of the cell. The cytoplasm is voluminous and in certain places appears granular.

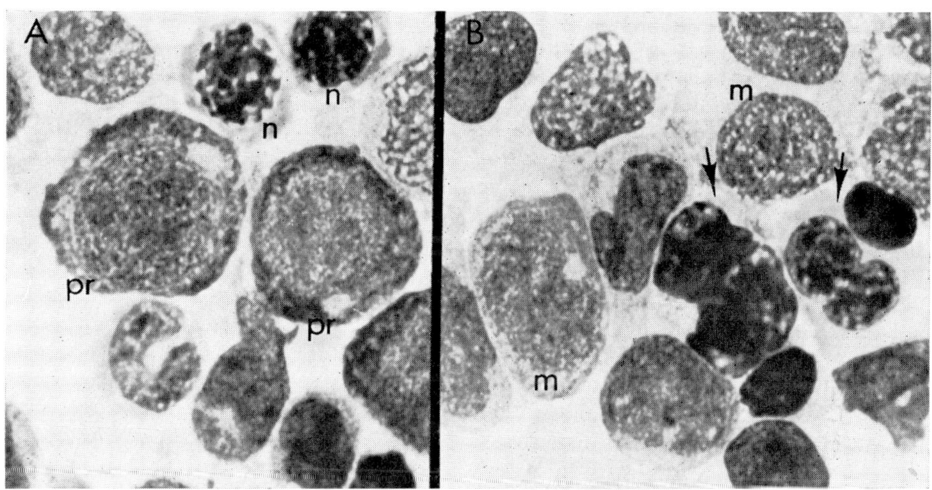

Figure 27. Erythroid abnormalities in myelomonocytic leukemia.

(A) Hyperplasia of proerythroblasts (pr) commonly seen in this type of leukemia, especially the subacute variety. Megaloblastoid intermediate macronormoblasts (n) can also be seen at the top of the photomicrograph.

(B) Two bizarre-appearing erythroid precursors (arrows) from a patient with subacute myelomonocytic leukemia. Multiple lobulations of the nucleus are seen, with nuclear appendages and a megaloblastoid type of chromatin pattern. Surrounding these cells are several neoplastic monocytes (m).

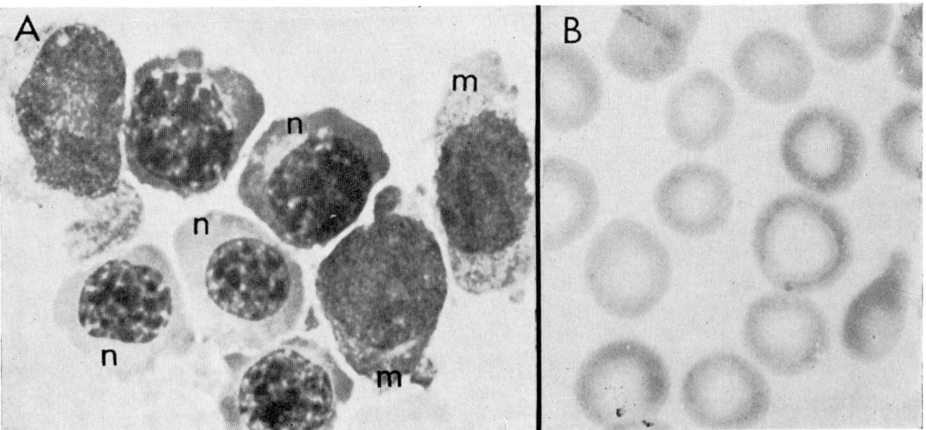

Figure 28. Erythroid abnormalities in subacute myelomonocytic leukemia.

(A) A group of megaloblastic intermediate macronormoblasts (n) surrounded by several neoplastic monocytes (m) containing multiple pseudopodia.

(B) The peripheral blood illustrates large macrocytic erythrocytes often found in the peripheral blood of patients with this disorder. The macrocytes presumably derive from the megaloblastoid erythroid precursors.

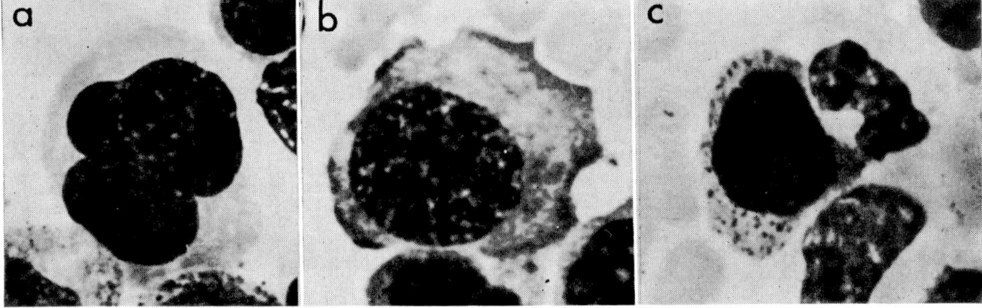

Figure 29. (a) Giant megaloblastoid intermediate macronormoblast with nucleus showing multiple lobulations.

(b) Large megaloblastoid intermediate macronormoblast with blocklike, fenestrated chromatin pattern and abundant, well-hemoglobinized cytoplasm.

(c) Late intermediate macronormoblast with megaloblastoid-type nuclear chromatin pattern and coarse cytoplasmic basophilic stippling.

by Beattie et al. and by Sinn and Dick appear to conform to our description of subacute myelomonocytic leukemia. Broun (37) has described "chronic erythromonocytic leukemia" in which disorders of erythropoiesis coincident with monocytosis appear to have many of the features of subacute myelomonocytic leukemia as described earlier. Other cases of "chronic" monocytic leukemia possessing features suggestive of subacute myelomonocytic leukemia have been described by Doan and Wiseman, (76) DiGuglielmo et al., (74) Rohkramer, (231)

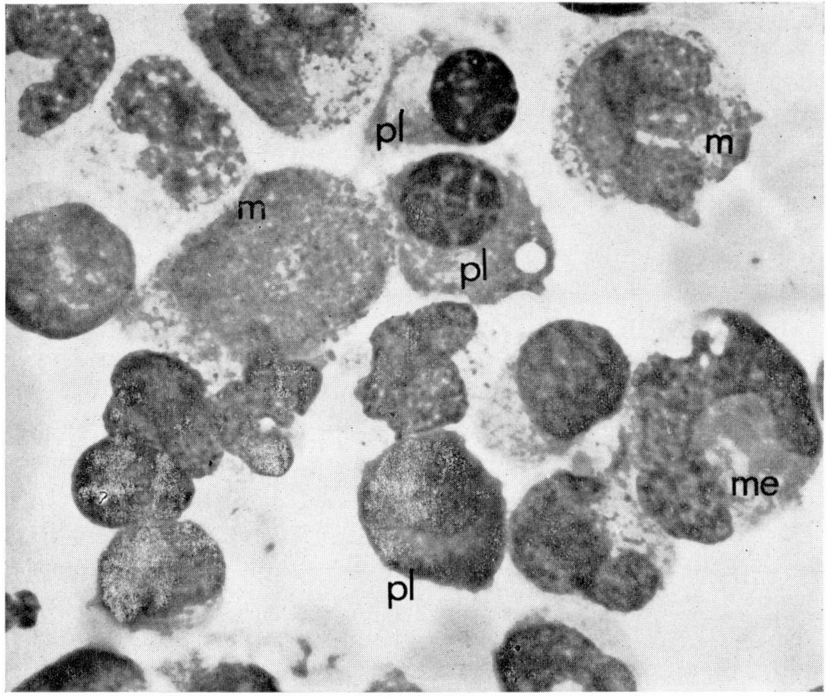

Figure 30. Plasmacytosis in subacute myelomonocytic leukemia. Increased numbers of mature-appearing plasma cells (pl) are commonly observed in this disorder. Neoplastic monocytes (m) and aberrant-appearing metamyelocytes (me) can also be seen surrounding the plasma cells.

Jacobsen, (134) Marchal et al., (163) Osgood, (205) Rappoport and Kugel, (218) Orr, (203) Pretlow (215) and Whitby and Christie. (299)

Preleukemia

At least some of the cases reported as "preleukemia" appear to conform to what we term subacute myelomonocytic leukemia. In the 1950's, several investigators became aware of a group of disorders which were frequently characterized by splenomegaly, pancytopenia and refractory anemia. This combination of findings often seemed to be the forerunner of acute leukemia, usually of the myeloblastic type. Block et al. in 1953 (26) described such cases as "preleukemic human acute leukemia" and noted that many of these cases demonstrated panmyelosis. In their study, other cases compatible with the diagnosis of "preleukemia" were characterized by aplastic anemia. In those with panmyelosis showing disturbances in granulopoiesis (maturation arrest) and erythropoiesis (extreme hyperplasia), normoblastemia was a frequent finding. Block et al. mention that at the time immature cells began to appear in the peripheral blood of their patients, "large numbers of monocytes" were seen. These authors further state that since there was some difficulty in distinguishing monocytes from myelocytes and metamyelocytes, "it will be impossible to determine whether the monocytosis seen is actual because of confusion of this cell type with the myelocytes." Many of the features described by Block et al. as being typical of "preleukemia" appear similar to those seen in what we term subacute myelomonocytic leukemia.

In 1954 Meacham and Weisberger (178) described atypical early manifestations of acute leukemia. They noted that several of their patients had macrocytic anemia, splenomegaly and monocytosis prior to the development of acute leukemia. It is not clear whether some of these acute leukemias were of the myelomonocytic or histiomonocytic types. Several of the cases described by Meacham and Weisberger are compatible with the diagnosis of subacute myelomonocytic leukemia.

In an investigation of atypical leukemias, Blair et al. (25) stated that none of the marrows of the patients in their study were diagnostic of acute leukemia. However, the majority of patients had monocytosis, normoblastemia, marrow hypercellularity, erythroid hyperplasia with qualitative abnormalities including megaloblastoid forms, the acquired Pelger-Huet anomaly (71) and poorly granulated polymorphonuclear leukocytes. Two of the patients had splenomegaly and all of them subsequently developed acute leukemia. The possibility exists that some of these patients may have had subacute myelomonocytic leukemia. The patients described by Blair et al. (25) appear to differ from those described by Rheingold et al. (224) as having "smouldering acute leukemia."

There have been several recent studies in patients with the diagnosis of "preleukemia" characterized by hyperplastic bone marrows which indicate a neoplastic character to "preleukemia" prior to the development of acute leukemia. Rowley et al. (238) described several patients with the diagnosis of preleukemia in whom chromosomal studies demonstrated a number of abnormalities including aneuploidy of group C chromosomes. In a study of chromosomal abnormalities in patients with preleukemia, Nowell (200) found that five of seven patients with preleukemia and chromosomal abnormalities died of acute leukemia within three months. He felt that a positive chromosomal study demonstrating various types of aberrations signified the imminent development of acute leukemia.

More recently, Greenburg et al. (114) have studied the granulocytic colony-forming capacity in patients with the diagnosis of preleukemia.

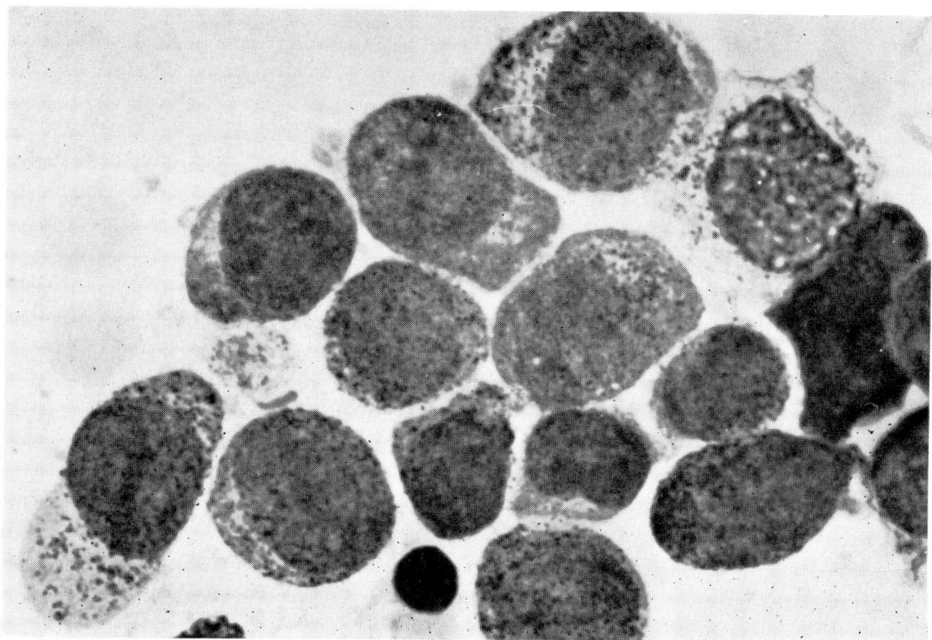

Figure 33. A cluster of leukemic blasts from a patient with acute myelomonocytic leukemia. Many of the blasts have monocytoid-appearing nuclei with prominent nucleoli. Neutrophilic-type granules are present in the abundant cytoplasm.

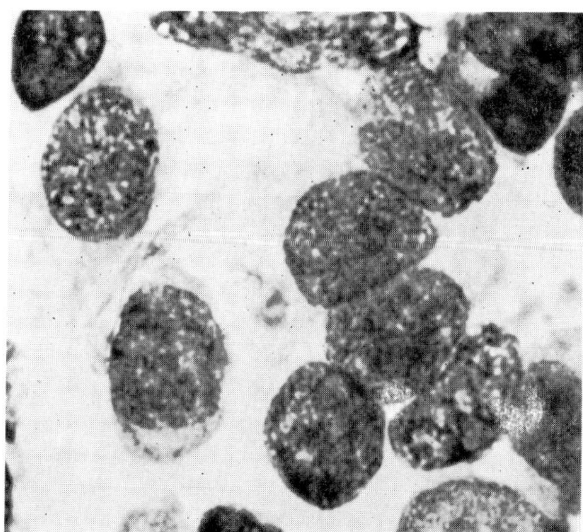

Figure 34. A group of reticulum cells, some of which have monocytoid nuclei, appear in a syncytial arrangement.

Granulocyte precursors are reduced and many of them show aberrant and sometimes monocytoid nuclei (Fig. 22). Megakaryocytes are reduced and may show bizarre-appearing nuclei (Fig. 26).

The electron microscopic appearance of leukemic blasts in acute myelomonocytic leukemia has been described by Hayhoe and Cawley, (121) Freeman and Journey (102) and Mori and Lennert. (190) Leukemic cells in Epon-embedded sections of peripheral blood vary somewhat in morphology from case to case. Some cells have nuclei which are very irregular in shape, while other cells have indented or bean-shaped nuclei (Fig. 35). Ultrastructurally, the leukemic cells from the peripheral blood of two patients with acute myelomonocytic leukemia (Figs. 36-43) generally have a relatively smooth surface, although some cells have short irregular cytoplasmic projec-

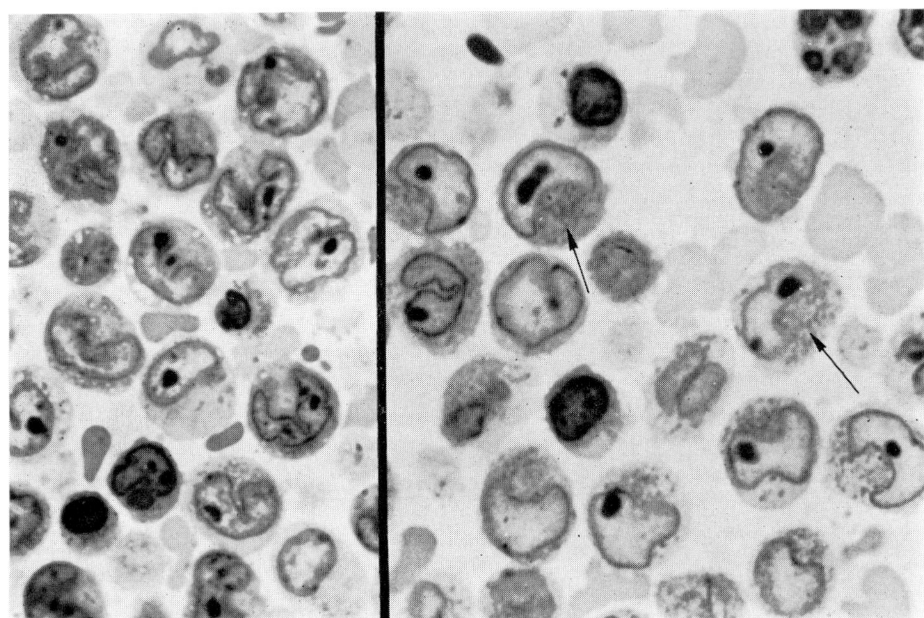

Figure 35. *(left)* A one-micron section of the peripheral blood of a patient with acute myelomonocytic leukemia. The leukemic cells have a slightly irregular cytoplasmic surface. The nuclei of most cells are very irregular in shape and contain one or sometimes two prominent nucleoli. A moderate to ample amount of cytoplasm is present.

(right). One-micron-thick section of cells from the peripheral blood of a patient with acute myelomonocytic leukemia. The leukemic cells are characterized by a small to moderate amount of cytoplasm, containing numerous small, dense structures (arrows), which correspond to mitochondria seen ultrastructurally. In many cells, these dense structures are polarized in the cytoplasm, and they are located in a shallow nuclear indentation. The nuclei are large, mostly indented, and contain little clumped chromatin. Some cells contain eccentrically placed nuclei with more aggregated chromatin. A prominent, large, round or elongated nucleolus is seen in most of the cells.

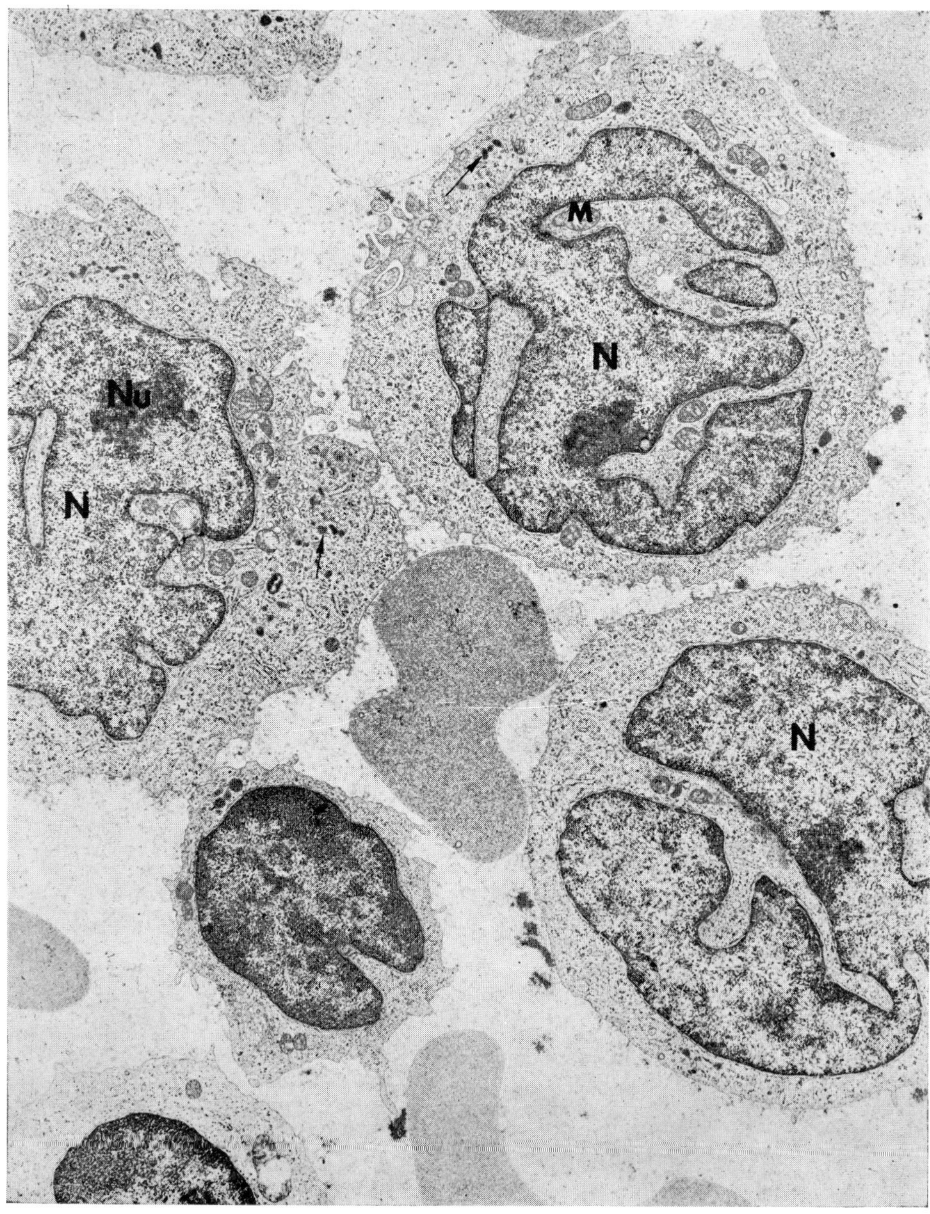

Figure 36. Leukemic cells from the peripheral blood of a patient with acute myelo-monocytic leukemia. The nuclei (N) of the cells are very irregular in shape. Heterochromatin is seen mostly at the periphery of the nucleus. Nucleoli (Nu) are prominent. The cytoplasm contains numerous polyribosomes and monoribosomes, few to moderate numbers of segments of granular endoplasmic reticulum, oval mitochondria (M) and few small dense granules (arrows).

tions. Many cells have extremely irregular nuclei (Fig. 36). These nuclei have a small to moderate amount of aggregated granular chromatin under the nuclear membrane. Nucleoli are seen in most cells. Nuclei of other cells are less irregular or have an indentation (Figs. 37-39). These nuclei have very little aggregated chromatin and contain large prominent nucleoli. Nuclear blebs and bridges are seen in some cells (Fig. 40a). A few cells which belong to the granulocytic series have many granules both of the azurophil (nonspecific) and specific types (Fig. 40b). The cytoplasm of some cells contains a moderate number of mitochondria randomly scattered throughout, while in other cells mitochondria are polarized in the cytoplasm of the nuclear concavity (Fig. 41). There are many polyribosomes (Fig. 42) and monoribosomes, and short segments of endoplasmic reticulum, and many cells have a fairly well-developed Golgi complex. Centrioles are seen in some cells (Fig. 42). Many cells are devoid of granules, while others have relatively few small, dense granules. Occasional cells contain bundles of microtubules in the perinuclear cytoplasm (Fig. 37). In a few cells, lipid bodies are present in the cytoplasm (Fig. 43).

Acute Histiomonocytic Leukemia (Schilling-Type)

In 1913, Reschad and Schilling-Torgau (221) described the first case of monocytic leukemia in a thirty-three-year-old mason with gingivitis, purpura, anemia, and increased numbers of "splenocytes" in his peripheral blood. These "splenocytes" were described as

almost typical large mononuclear cells and transition forms. . . they showed very fine azurophilic granulations of their endoplasm and a nucleus consisting of fine fibers and pale-staining characteristics and with a tendency to polymorphia; rarely one could see very small nucleoli. The protoplasm was always relatively large; nucleus and protoplasm rather large in comparison with other blood cells. The oxidase reaction was always negative. The cells which were very similar to the transition forms showed an atypical tendency to lobulation of the nucleus, some of which had bizarre configuration; often a surprisingly clear segregation in the ectoplasm and fine granulated endoplasm; frequent formation of serrated pseudopodia. Many cells showed central vacuoles or very large spherical formations with distinct centrosomes.

Plate 5 represents a reproduction of these "splenocytes" (monocytes) from the peripheral blood of this patient, as published subsequently by Schilling in 1929. (252)

Reschad and Schilling did not propose a separate reticuloendothelial stem cell for the monocyte in their 1913 publication. In 1926, Schilling (251) proposed his "trialistic theory" of blood formation, although he had suggested in 1912 (253) that the monocyte represented a cellular

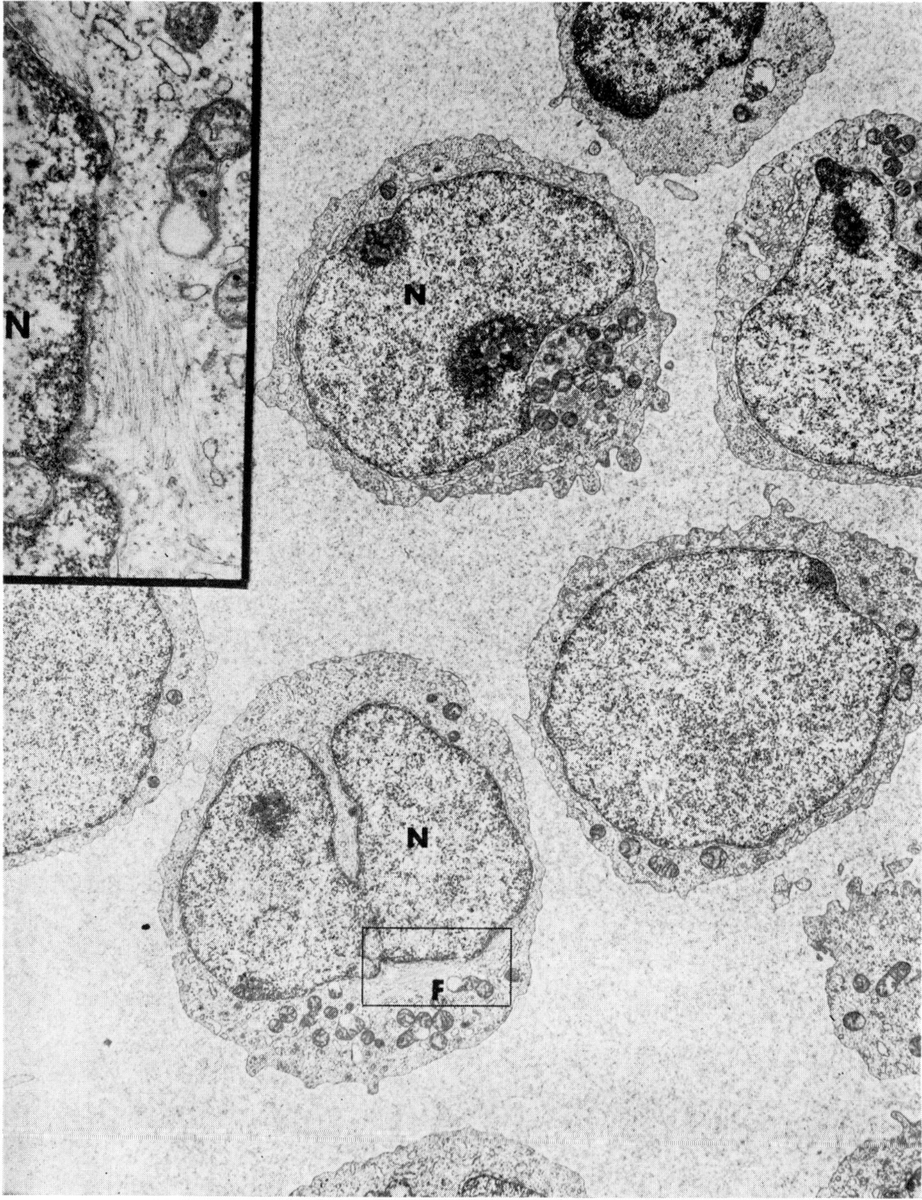

Figure 37. Leukemic cells from a patient with acute myelomonocytic leukemia. The primitive cells have smooth or irregularly contoured cytoplasm containing large, irregularly shaped, indented or oval nuclei (N). There is little clumping of chromatin, and one or two prominent nucleoli are seen. Mitochondria are polarized in one part of the cytoplasm. The cell with the clefted nucleus contains a prominent band of microfibrils in the perinuclear cytoplasm. *Inset* Higher magnification of the area with the rectangle showing a part of the nucleus (N) and bundles of microfibrils in the adjacent cytoplasm.

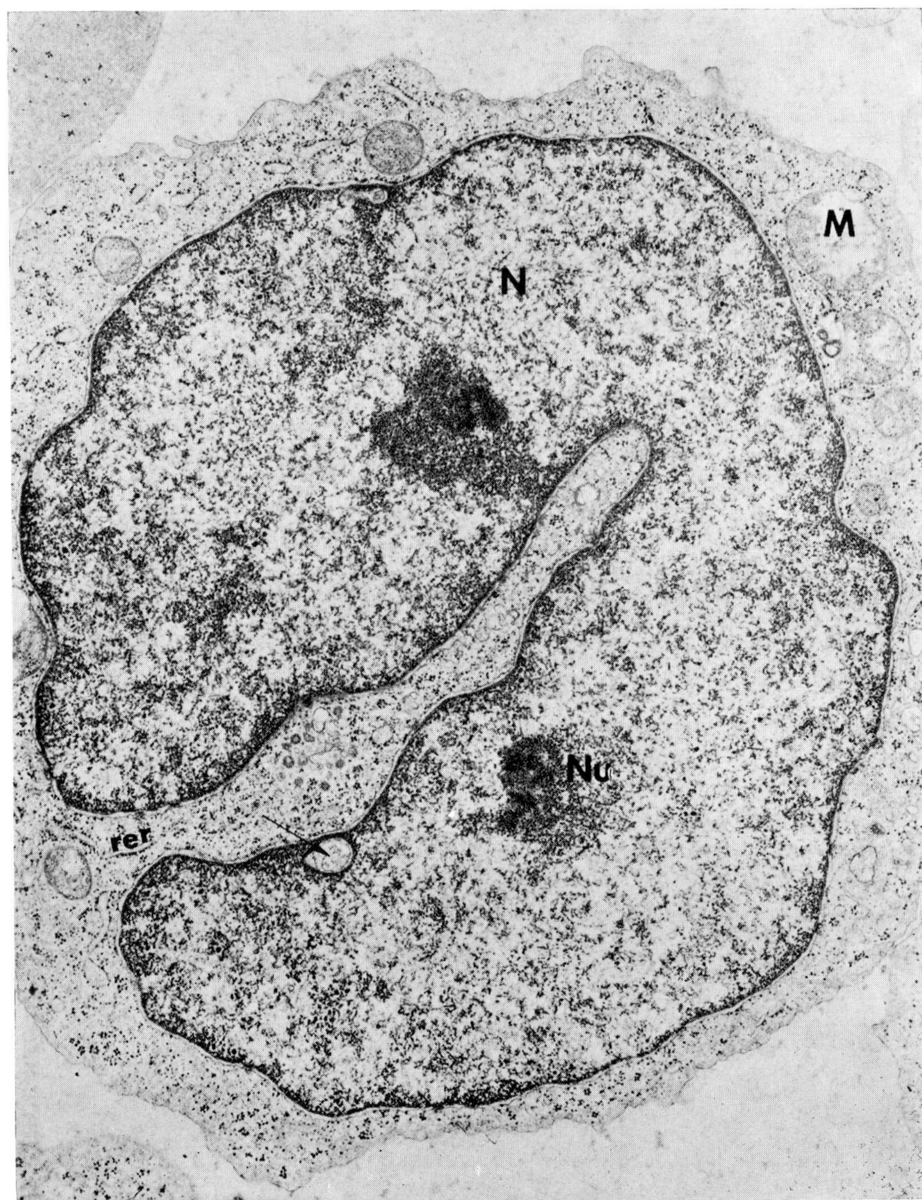

Figure 38. A leukemic cell with a horseshoe-shaped nucleus (N) containing a moderate amount of heterochromatin and a nucleolus (Nu) in each nuclear lobe. A small inclusion of cytoplasm is seen in the nucleus (arrow). The cytoplasm contains monoribosomes, polyribosomes, short segments of rough endoplasmic reticulum (rer) and a few mitochondria (M).

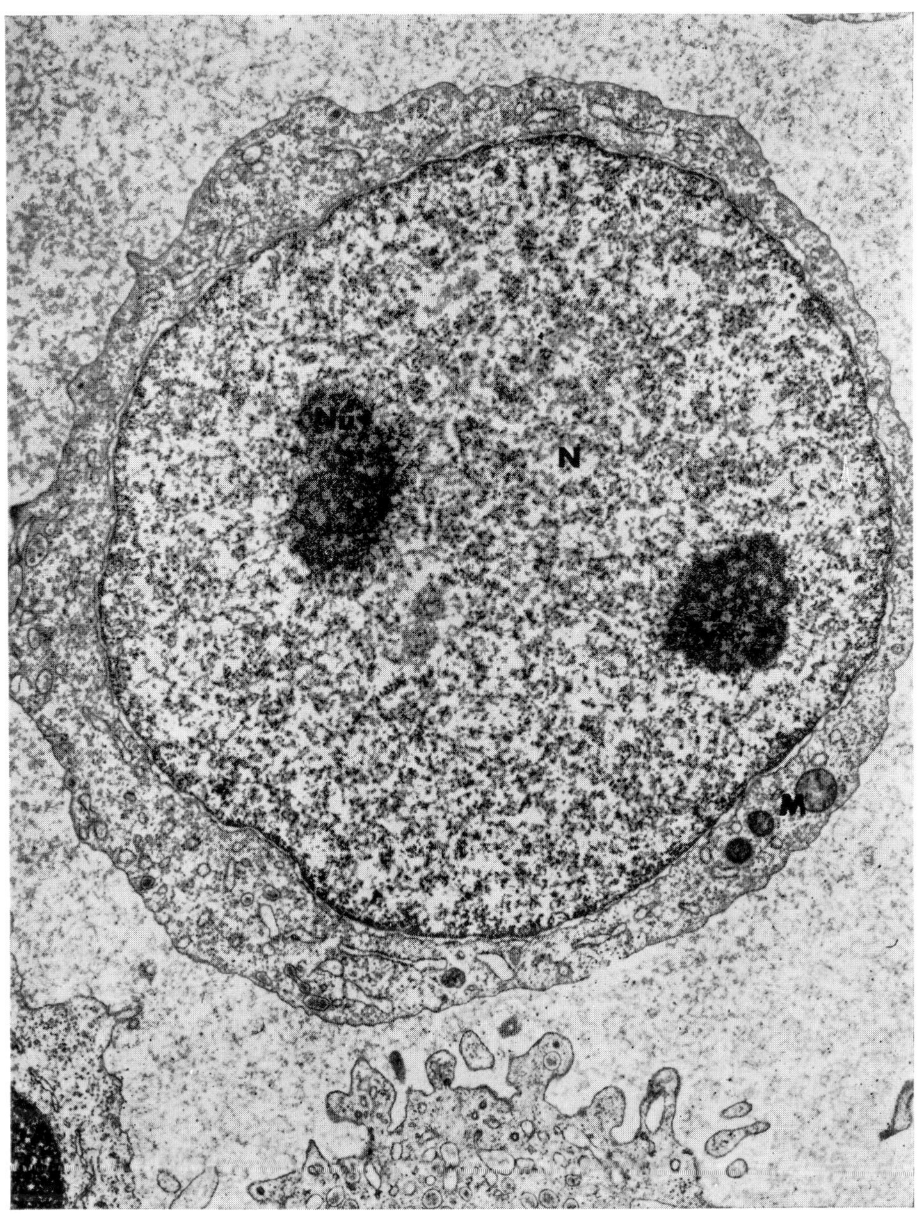

Figure 39. A cell from the peripheral blood of a patient with acute myelomonocytic leukemia. The surface of the leukemic cell is relatively smooth. The nucleus (N) is large and has practically no clumping of chromatin. Two large, prominent nucleoli (Nu) are present. The small amount of cytoplasm is devoid of granules, contains few mitrochondria and a moderate number of ribosomes scattered throughout. A few membranes of granular endoplasmic reticulum and small vacuoles are present. Some of these appear to be granules, which contain slightly electron-dense amorphous material surrounded by an electron-lucent zone.

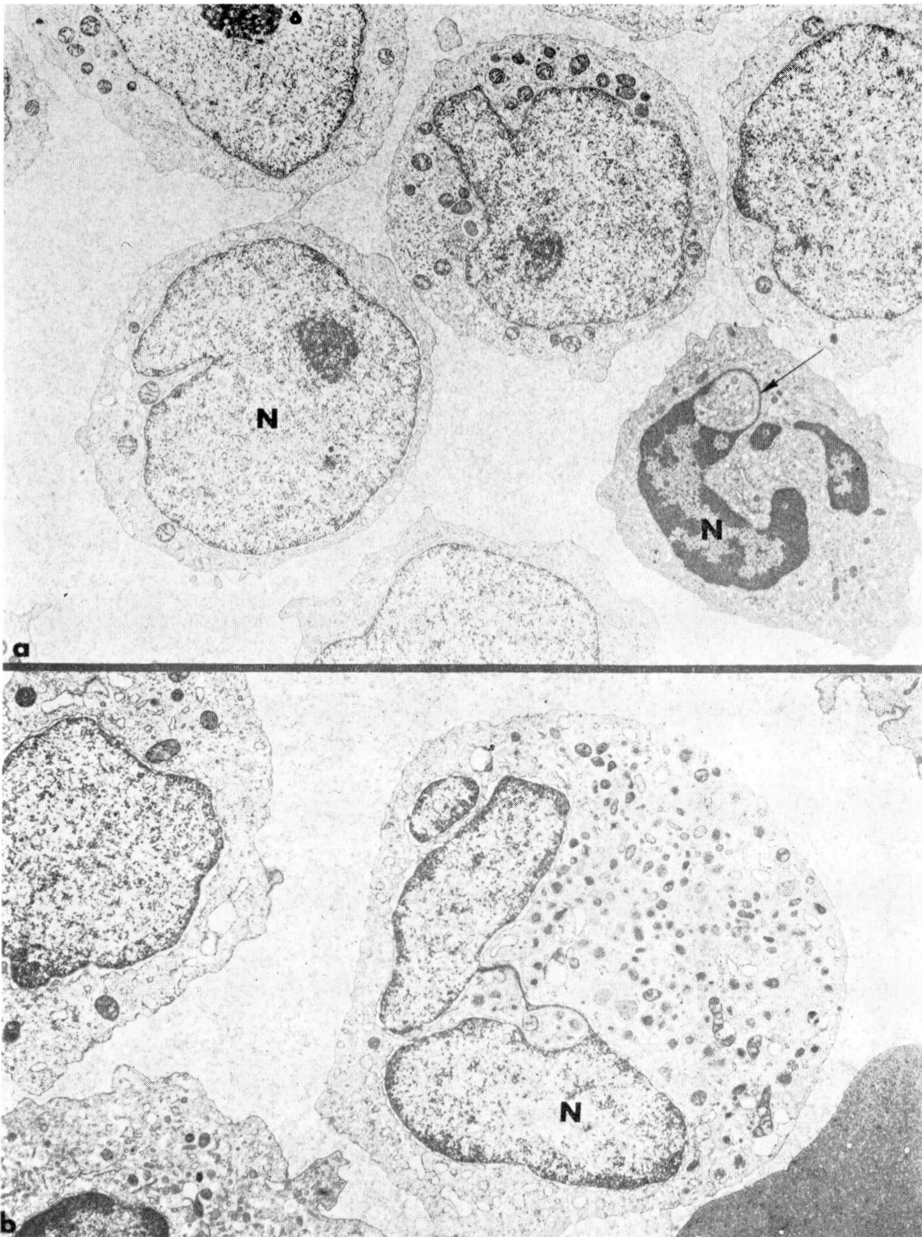

Figure 40. Leukemic cells from a case of acute myelomonocytic leukemia. (a) The cells appear immature with little aggregation of nuclear chromatin and contain prominent nucleoli. One cell has considerable condensation of chromatin and has a nuclear bleb (arrow). (b) A granulocytic leukemic cell with two large nuclear lobes connected by a nuclear bridge. The cytoplasm contains both primary (azurophil) and secondary granules in the cytoplasm.

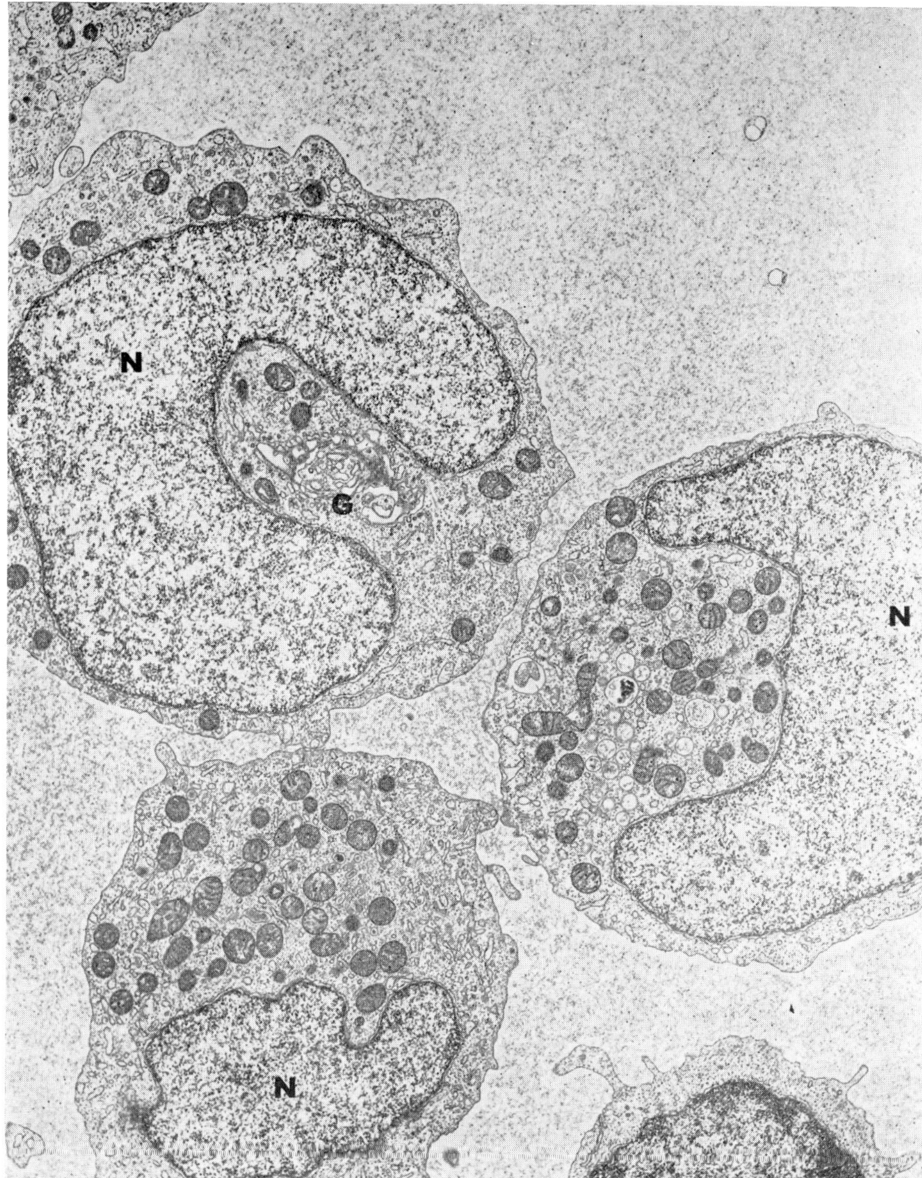

Figure 41. Three leukemic cells from a patient with acute myelomonocytic leukemia. The nuclei (N) are indented and mitochondria are polarized in the cytoplasm of the nuclear concavity. A Golgi (G) complex is seen in this area of the cytoplasm in one of the cells.

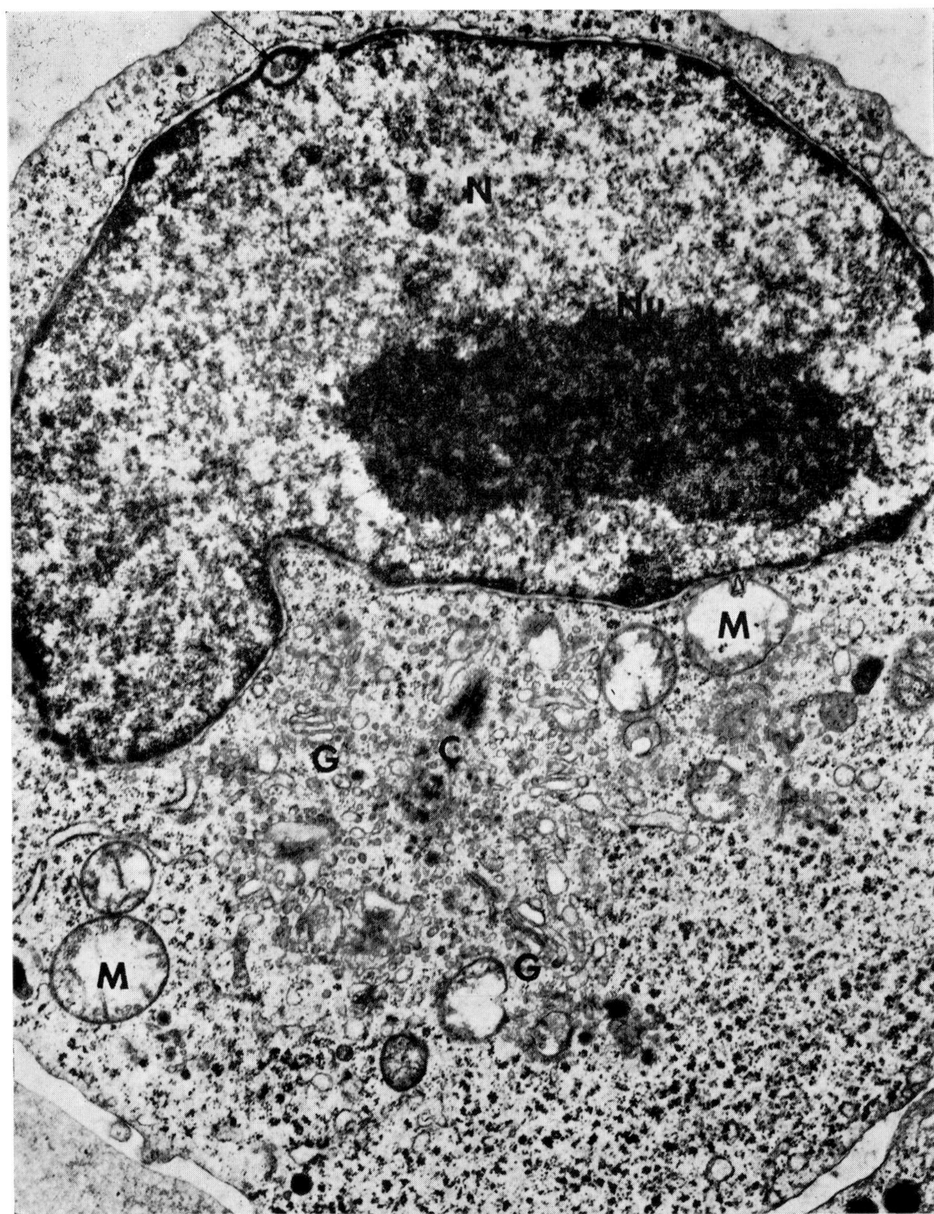

Figure 42. A leukemic cell with an indented nucleus (N) containing a large nucleolus (Nu). Numerous polyribosomes are seen in the cytoplasm of the nuclear concavity. (Arrow) cytoplasmic inclusion in the nucleus; (M) mitochondria.

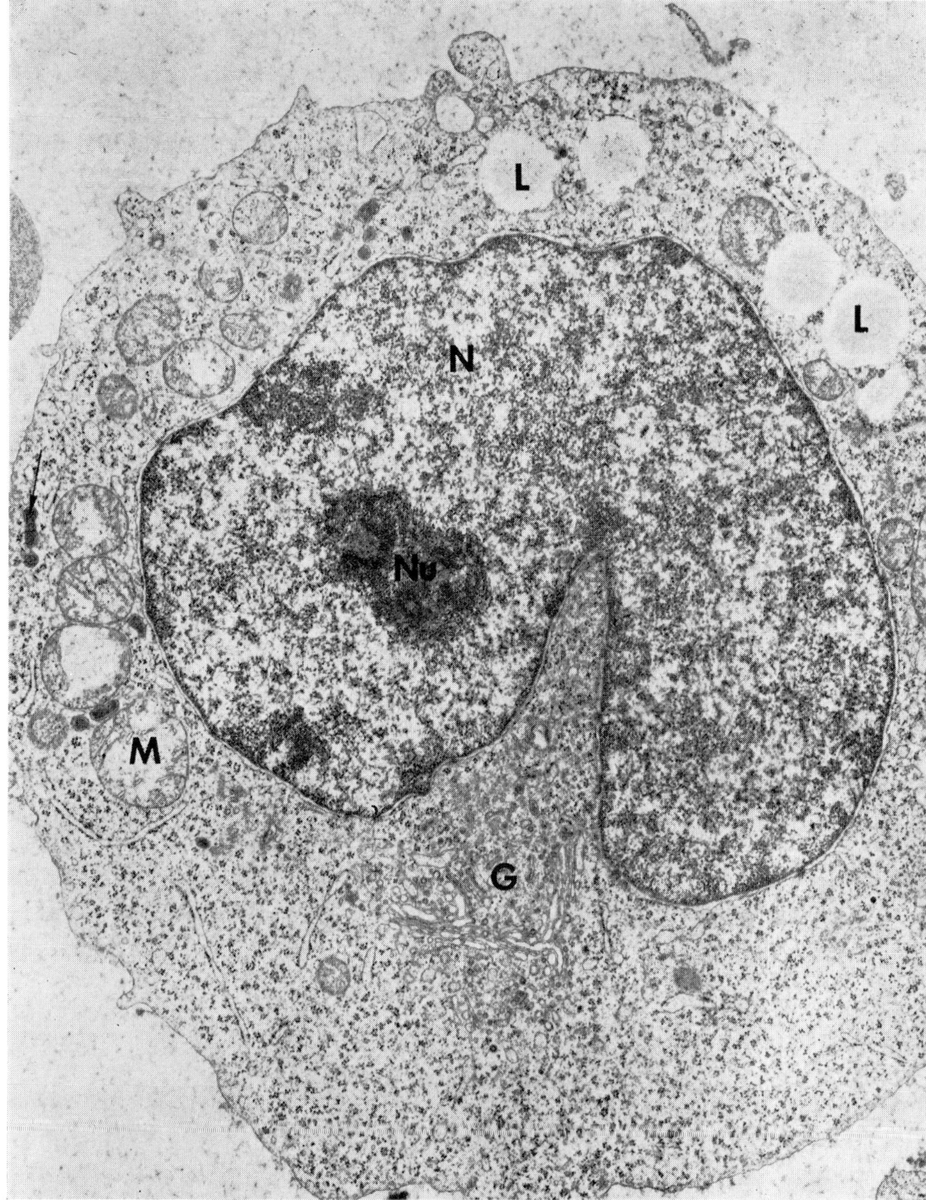

Figure 43. A leukemic cell with an indented nucleus (N) containing a moderate amount of heterochromatin and a prominent nucleolus (Nu). In addition to many polyribosomes, mitochondria (M), short segments of rough endoplasmic reticulum, a Golgi complex (G) and rare small electron-dense granules (arrow), the cytoplasm also contains lipid bodies (L).

system separate from lymphoid and myeloid cells. Fleischmann (95) reported the second case of monocytic leukemia in 1915. In the American literature, the first case of monocytic leukemia was described by Rosenthal in 1921 (233) as an atypical case of leukemia. Numerous other publications of cases of monocytic leukemia ensued (10,14,23, 30,43,48,49,56,65,89,97,100,134,135,149,162,163,184, 185, 205, 250, 267, 281,297,298,299)

The clinical presentation of this disease is similar to that seen in acute myelomonocytic leukemia, except that hyperplasia of the gums along with splenomegaly are more constant features in acute histiomonocytic leukemia. The gingival hypertrophy may be spectacular as seen in Figure 44, and skin manifestations in the form of violaceous maculopapular lesions are common and resemble those seen in acute myelomonocytic leukemia (Figure 32).

The peripheral white count is generally elevated but on occasion may be low or normal. The patient is usually anemic at the time of diagnosis, and thrombocytopenia is generally present.

The peripheral blood film shows neoplastic monocytes which may appear different from those seen in acute myelomonocytic leukemia (Plate 6). These monocytes are large cells measuring up to 50 μ in

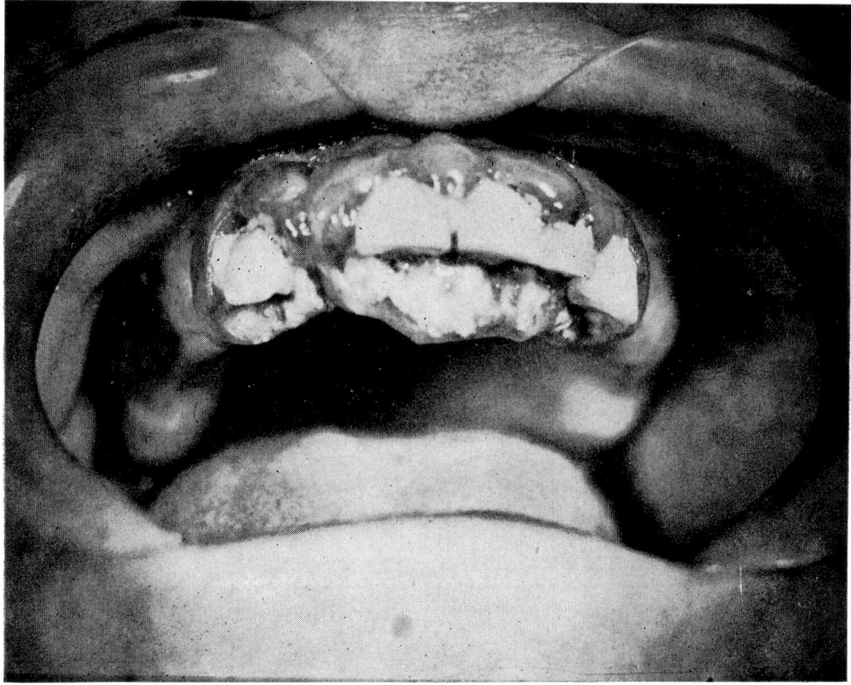

Figure 44. Striking gingival hyperplasia in a patient with acute histiomonocytic leukemia.

diameter in some cases. The cell appears to be fluid, often assuming an elongated shape with a long cytoplasmic "tail." Multiple pseudopodia are common, and the gray-blue cytoplasm may have abundant nonspecific azurophil and pink granules (Plates 6,7; Fig. 45). There may be both histiomonoblasts with a large oval nucleus, multiple nucleoli and scant cytoplasm, and histiomonocytes with more abundant cytoplasm and a nucleus with elaborate nuclear foldings and delicate chromatin strands. Circulating hemohistiocytes and hemohistioblasts are common. The erythrocytes may show considerable anisocytosis and poikilocytosis, but macrocytes, as seen in subacute and acute myelomonocytic leukemia, are less common.

A typical bone marrow from a patient with acute histiomonocytic leukemia is illustrated in Plate 6 and Figure 45. Numerous histiomonoblasts with features described above are present. Granulocytes and erythroid precursors are reduced in number and the latter generally

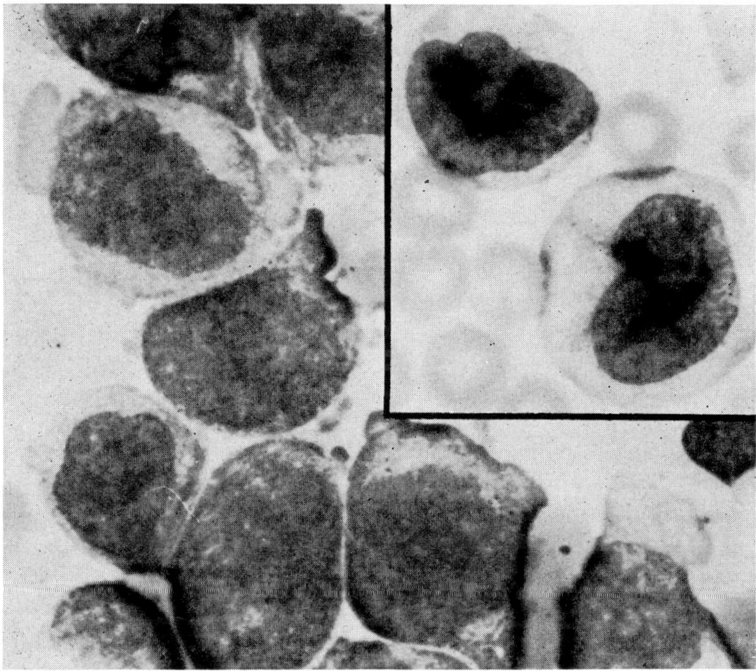

Figure 45. Acute histiomonocytic leukemia. The larger portion of the composite shows histiomonoblasts from the bone marrow. Multiple nuclear lobulations and infoldings and prominent nucleoli can be seen. The cytoplasm is gray-blue in color and shows several clear ectoplasmic pseudopodia and nonspecific granules. The inset at the upper right shows two histiomonocytes from the peripheral blood of this patient. The nuclear chromatin is fine, and the nuclear lobulations appear to overlie one another. The cytoplasm is clear, staining blue-gray, and contains numerous nonspecific dust-like granules.

show normoblastic maturation. Cytoplasmic shedding by blasts is common. Hyperplasia of hemohistiocytes and hemohistioblasts is often striking, and many of these cells have indentations or foldings of their nuclei (Fig. 46).

Epon-embedded sections of peripheral blood from a patient with acute histiomonocytic leukemia show leukemic cells with abundant cytoplasm. The large nuclei are vesicular and contain a single large nucleolus or several small nucleoli (Fig. 47).

Freeman and Journey (102) and Hayhoe and Cawley (120) have described the electron microscopic appearance of leukemic blasts in histiomonocytic leukemia. Figures 48 to 51 illustrate leukemic cells from a patient with acute histiomonocytic leukemia as viewed under the electron microscope. The surface is irregularly contoured due to the presence of depressions and broad cytoplasmic projections (Fig. 48). Many of the cytoplasmic projections are devoid of organelles other than ribosomes while some of the projections contain in addition, occasional dense granules, rough endoplasmic reticulum, vacuoles and vesicles. The nuclei of the leukemic cells are generally irregular or bean shaped (Figs. 48-50). The chromatin is mostly light-staining, while at the periphery of the nucleus, small amounts of granular clumped chromatin is visible. Most cells contain a single nucleolus, and some nuclei have two. Ten to twenty round or oval mitochondria are seen in most cells. Well-formed Golgi complexes may be present and centrioles are seen in a small percentage of cells. Small oval, round or elongated electron-dense granules are noted in most cells. Occasional small granules appear in the region of the Golgi vesicles. The latter may be early, newly formed granules. Occasional small granules have a central dense core surrounded by a more electron-opaque zone. A moderate number of membranes of rough endoplasmic reticulum with slightly dilated cisternae are scattered within the cytoplasm, and a number of these organelles may be grouped in one area of cytoplasm. Some polyribosomes are seen throughout the cytoplasm. Vacuoles and vesicles are present near the surface of the cell and within cytoplasmic projections of the cell. Bundles of microfibrils, especially in the perinuclear part of the cytoplasm were seen in many leukemic cells (Figs. 49,50). These microfibrils appeared to be identical to those seen in normal monocytes from the peripheral blood. Splitting of bundles of microfibrils (Fig. 50) with incorporation of mitochondria, membranes of rough endoplasmic reticulum and ribosomes, however, was not seen in normal monocytes. Occasional bundles or groups of microfibrils were seen in the more peripheral parts of the cytoplasm. Several leukemic cells also had cytoplasmic inclusions composed of what appeared to be denser aggregates of

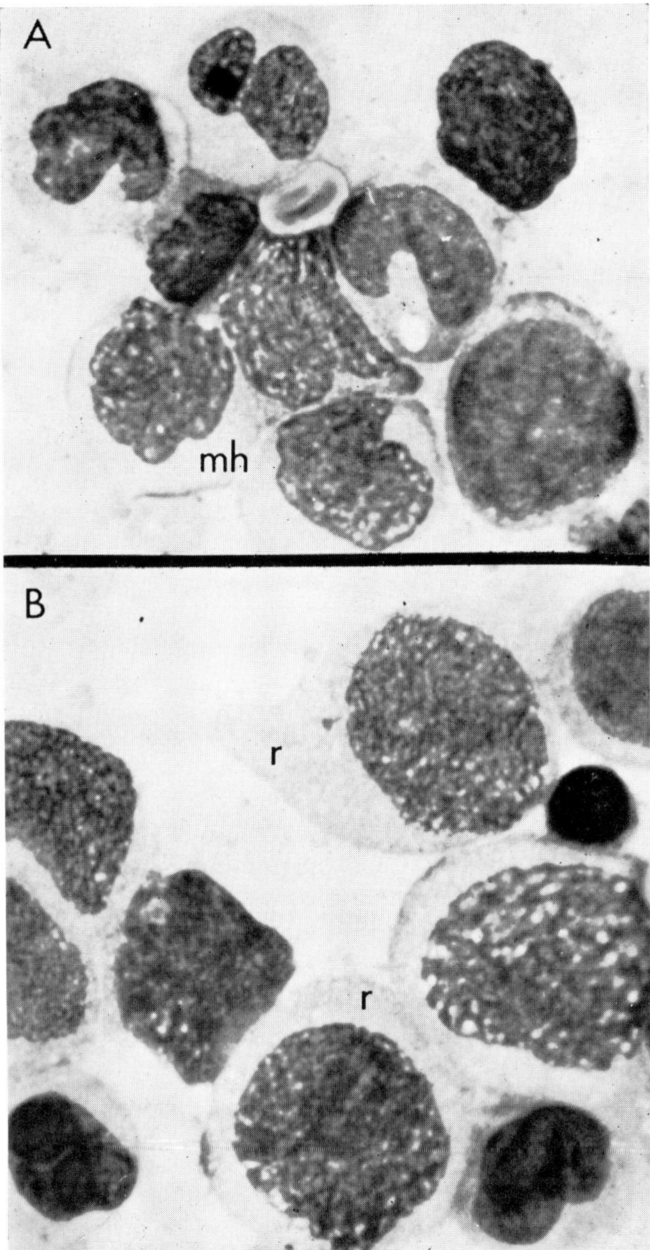

Figure 46. Hemohistiocytic and reticulum cell abnormalities in histiomonocytic leukemias.

(A) Monocytoid hemohistioblasts (mh) in a patient with acute histiomonocytic leukemia.

(B) Unusually large, neoplastic-appearing reticulum cells (r), some of which have abundant cytoplasm, from another patient with acute histiomonocytic leukemia.

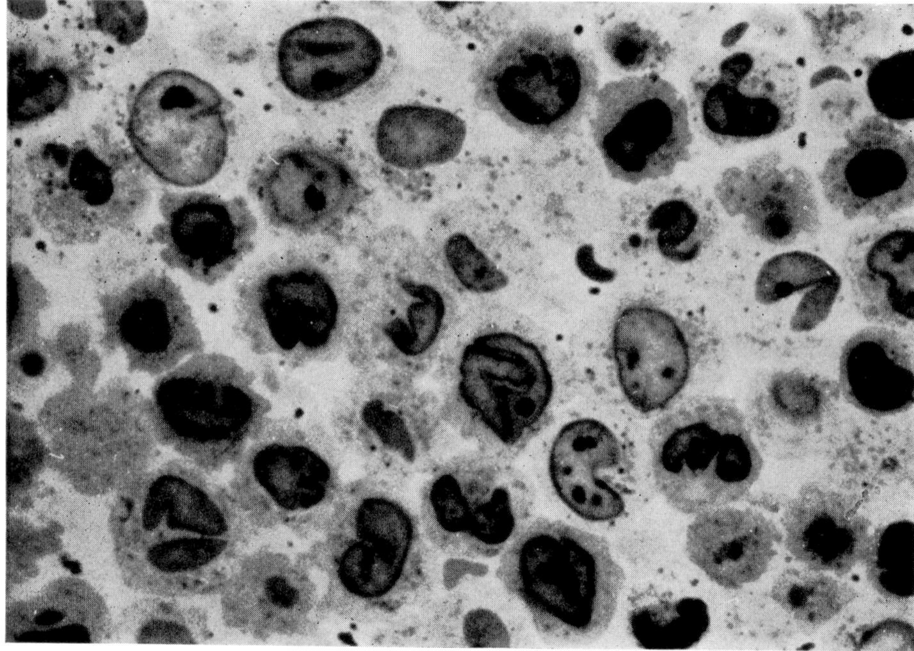

Figure 47. One-micron-thick section of peripheral blood from a patient with histiomonocytic leukemia. The leukemic cells have abundant cytoplasm which has an irregular surface and contains scattered dense structures. The nuclei are large, vesicular and irregular and often contain deep clefts or indentations or else are horseshoe shaped. A single, large nucleolus or several smaller nucleoli are present in many cells.

fibrils coursing about an area of the nucleus (Fig. 51).

Ultrastructurally, the cells in histiomonocytic leukemia resemble monocytes from the peripheral blood of healthy individuals. Both monocytes and histiomonocytic leukemic cells often have horseshoe-shaped nuclei, cytoplasmic bundles of microfibrils around the nucleus and small electron granules. The leukemic cells appeared to have less heterochromatin in their nuclei than normal monocytes, and the microfibrils in the cytoplasm of leukemic cells sometimes appear to take an aberrant course and surround organelles. Inclusions are occasionally seen in the cytoplasm of leukemic cells but are not seen in monocytes from healthy individuals.

Treatment of Monocytic Leukemias

A number of single and multiple drug regimens (33,57,88,105,108, 148) have been developed for the treatment of monocytic leukemias. However, to date, none of these regimens has produced uniformly satisfactory results. Likewise, what constitutes a satisfactory maintenance program in those patients who have sustained a complete remission is currently an unresolved issue.

of the histiomonocytic and reticulum type have electron-dense granules which are absent or only rarely observed in hairy cells. The Golgi apparatus also appears to be better developed and more often seen in the histiomonocytic and reticulum cells. The ribosome-lamella complex has been described in the hairy cell and not in other leukemic cells.

Routine bone marrow aspirates from patients with hairy cell leukemia are usually very dilute. The difficulty encountered in obtaining a satisfactory marrow aspirate might be related to the hair-like processes on the surface of the cells which may interdigitate with those of neighboring hairy cells. A typical bone marrow aspirate from a patient with hairy cell leukemia is seen in Figure 52c. The marrow is largely replaced by neoplastic "lymphoreticular" cells. Bone marrow biopsies in these patients show patchy replacement of the normal architecture by cells which have indistinct cytoplasmic borders and are not closely packed together, as are the cells of lymphomas, but rather appear to be separated from one another (Fig. 58). Histologically, these cells are different from both reticulum cells and lymphocytes, although they resemble the latter cells more closely (Fig. 59). The nuclei are oval, some contain clefts, and there is a moderate

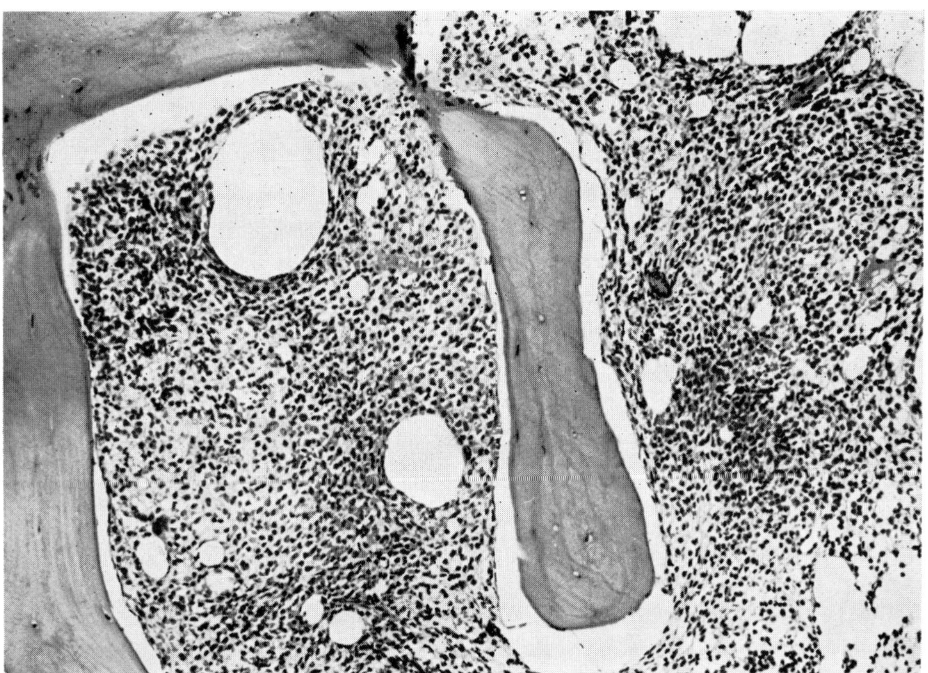

Figure 58. A bone marrow biopsy from a patient with hairy cell leukemia. The architecture of the marrow is replaced by a monotonous proliferation of "lymphoreticular" cells. Only a few fat spaces remain.

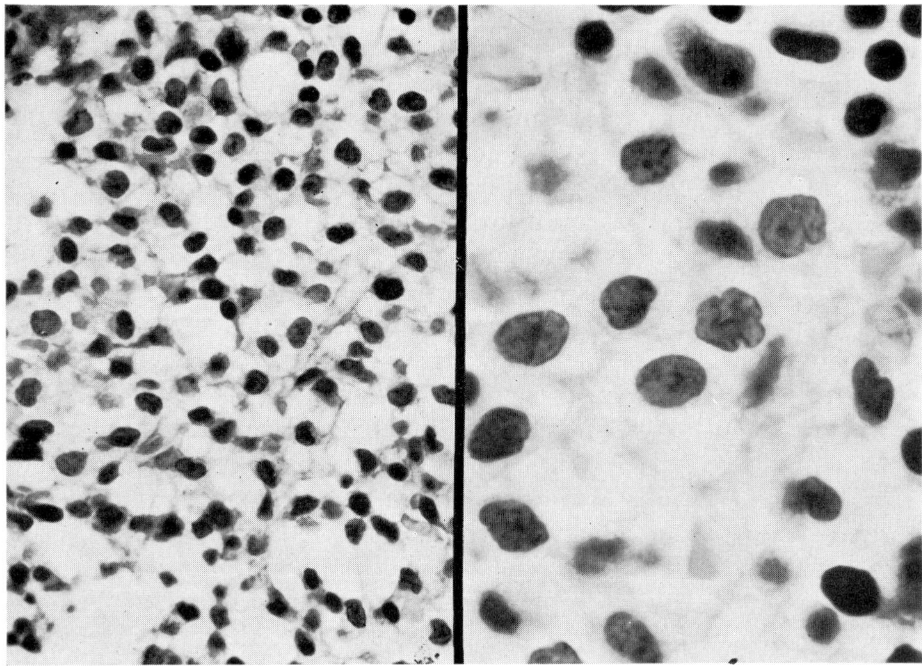

Figure 59. Higher magnification of hairy cells of Figure 58. *(left)* The leukemic cells have indistinct cytoplasmic borders and appear to lie separated from one another within the marrows. *(right)* The nuclei are oval shaped, some containing a cleft, and there appears to be considerable clumping of chromatin. Small nucleoli are seen in a few cells.

amount of chromatin aggregation throughout the nucleus. Reticulum stains of marrow biopsies show some condensation of reticulin fibers in the involved areas.

Leukemic Phase of Reticulum Cell Sarcoma

The term "reticulosarcoma" was introduced by Oberling (201) in 1928. The same or a similar type of neoplasm of the lymphoreticular system has been described under such names as "endothelioma of lymph nodes" by Ewing in 1913, (91) "reticulum cell lymphosarcoma" by Gohn and Roman in 1916, (111) "a malignant proliferation of lymph node reticuloendothelial tissue" by Goormaghtigh in 1925, (112) "retothelsarkom" by Roulet in 1930 (236) and 1932 (237) and reticulo-endotheliosis by Ritchie and Meyer (228) in 1936. In the American literature this neoplasm is now called "reticulum cell sarcoma" or "histiocytic lymphoma." (217) Entities such as aleukemic reticulosis (67) may represent variants of reticulum cell sarcoma.

In a small percentage of cases, reticulum cell sarcoma may have a leukemic phase in which the peripheral blood and bone marrow become flooded with neoplastic cells. (156,157,164,165,259,312) Clinically, most patients with leukemic reticulum cell sarcoma have hepatomegaly and splenomegaly. The splenomegaly is often massive. Peripheral lymphadenopathy may be absent or minimal, but abdominal masses often representing retroperitoneal and/or gastrointestinal involvement by reticulum cell sarcoma may be present. Central nervous system manifestations including cranial nerve palsies and paraplegias are also common. They usually represent involvement of the central nervous system with reticulum cell sarcoma or are secondary to intracranial hemorrhage due to thrombocytopenia.

Anemia which is normochromic and normocytic is usually present when the patient is leukemic. The white blood count may be low, normal or elevated, and is usually above 10,000 mm³. The majority of the cells are leukemic blasts. Thrombocytopenia and granulocytopenia may be seen. Granulocytic precursors, particularly metamyelocytes and juvenile forms, may be seen in the peripheral blood and may have an abnormal nuclear configuration. Aberrant-appearing monocytes and unusually large macrocytic erythrocytes may also occur.

Ohara et al. (202) performed cytokinetic studies in a patient with leukemic reticulum cell sarcoma. They found that the mean generation time of the labelled neoplastic reticulum cells after continuous infusion of tritium-labelled thymidine was six days. The duration of S was one day, G2 was five hours, M was two hours, and G1 was five days. A three-day infusion of cytosine arabinoside killed approximately half the reticulum sarcoma cells, but within nine days after stopping the drug, the remaining cells were proliferating at the same rate as the whole population of cells.

Of the three patients with leukemic reticulum cell sarcoma studied by Schnitzer and Kass, (259) all had biopsy-proven reticulum cell sarcoma before leukemic cells were discovered in the peripheral blood and bone marrow. One patient had a mixed, diffuse and nodular histologic pattern of reticulum cell sarcoma, the second patient a diffuse pattern and the third patient a nodular pattern (Figs. 60,61).

A spectrum of cell types may be seen in the peripheral blood in these cases of leukemic reticulum cell sarcoma, ranging from primitive reticulum cells to cells with monocytoid features and to cells that are morphologically indistinguishable from those seen in histiomonocytic leukemia. (259) The monocytic nature of some of these leukemic reticulum cells is further attested to by the presence of esterase activity when alpha-naphthyl acetate is used as the substrate. (259) This nonspecific esterase activity can be used as a marker for the identification of monocytes and histiocytes. (6,143,144,145,146,254,257, 307)

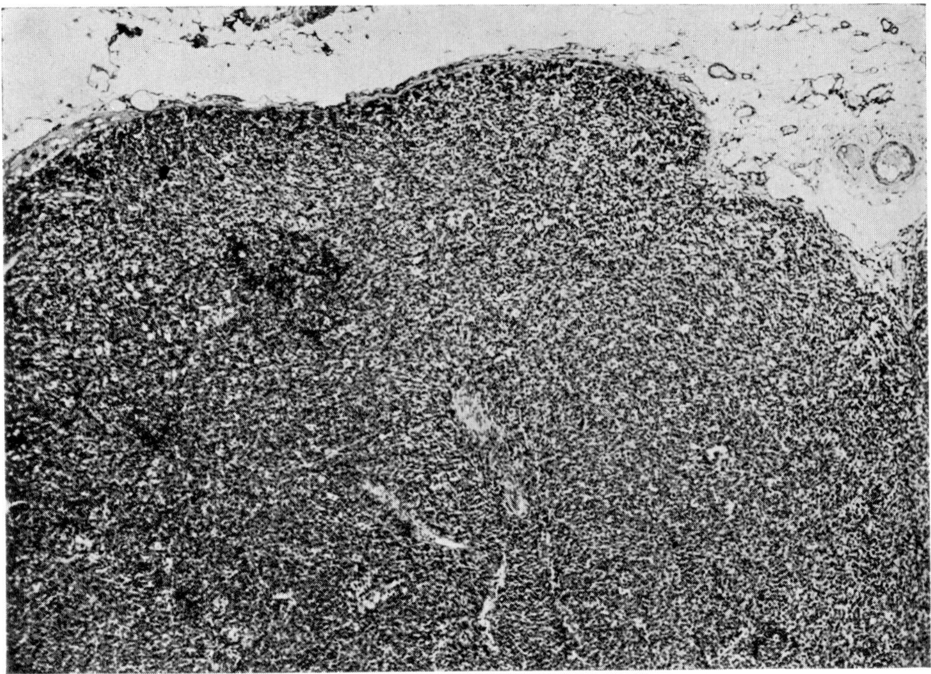

Figure 60. Biopsy of a lymph node from a patient with the histiocytic type of reticulum cell sarcoma that became leukemic. The normal nodal architecture is effaced by a diffuse proliferation of reticulum cells.

The variety of cytological types of leukemic cells from the peripheral blood and bone marrow of these three patients with leukemic reticulum cell sarcoma is illustrated in Plates 10-12. As seen in Plate 10, the neoplastic reticulum cells are large mononuclear cells with fine nuclear chromatin and an unusually prominent nucleolus. The cytoplasm is intensely basophilic and shows radial striations. Similar cells with many cytoplasmic vacuoles were found in large numbers (50 percent) in the bone marrow (Plate 10a). Cytologically, these particular cells (Plate 10b,c,d) strongly resemble those illustrated by Downey (Plate 9) as being typical of the cells seen in leukemic reticuloendotheliosis.

Epon-embedded sections of leukemic cells from the peripheral blood of this patient are characterized by large, slightly irregular or indented vesicular nuclei which have only a small amount of chromatin concentrated at their periphery (Fig. 62). Most of the nuclei contain a single, large and prominent nucleolus, while some nuclei have two smaller nucleoli. With higher magnification (Fig. 62b), small dense cytoplasmic structure concentrated mostly in one portion of the cytoplasm are seen to correspond to groups of mitochondria seen ultrastructurally.

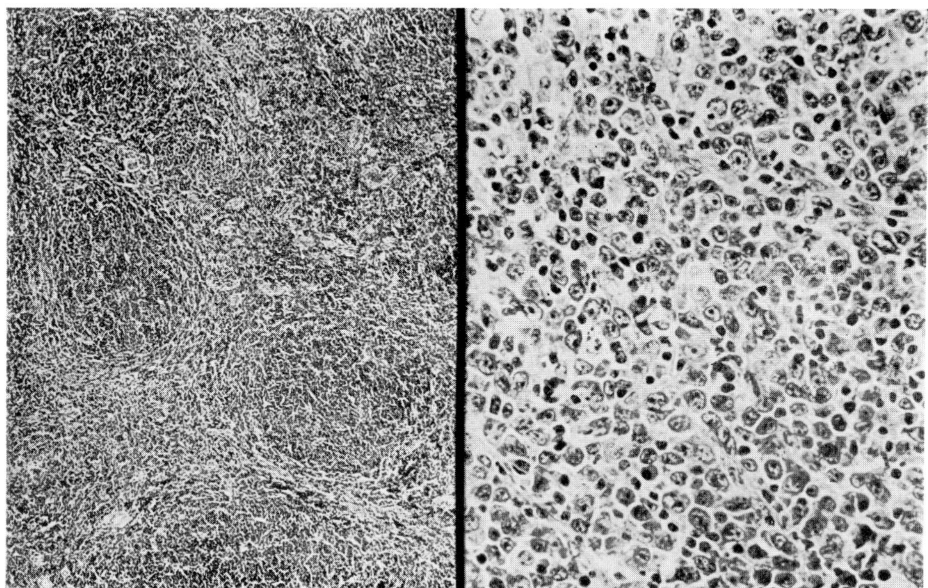

Figure 61. Lymph node biopsy from a patient with a histiocytic type of reticulum cell sarcoma (histiocytic lymphoma) that subsequently became leukemic. *(left)* The normal architecture of the lymph node is replaced by a proliferation of reticulum cells which are arranged in a nodular (follicular) pattern. *(right)* Higher magnification shows that the neoplastic reticulum cells have ample cytoplasm with large vesicular, oval nuclei in which a small amount of chromatin is present but only along the nuclear membrane. Most cells contain a single, large nucleolus, while others have two small nucleoli.

Electron microscopically, the surface of the leukemic reticulum cells is smooth, and only rarely is a microvillous projection of cytoplasm noted (Fig. 63). The leukemic cells have large, somewhat irregularly shaped or slightly indented nuclei which contain mostly light-staining euchromatin in the central portions and irregular areas of condensed granular heterochromatin distributed along the nuclear membrane (Fig. 63a). A large and prominent nucleolus was seen in almost all the cells, while a few nuclei contained two smaller nucleoli. The cytoplasm of many cells contained forty to fifty mitochondria grouped on one side of the nucleus, often in a nuclear concavity, with a few mitochondria randomly scattered throughout the cytoplasm. (Fig. 63a,b). The mitochondria varied considerably in size and shape (Fig. 63b), some large and irregular, and occasionally one with a dumbbell shape. One or more well-developed Golgi complexes were seen in many cells (Fig. 63c). Small Golgi vesicles, some containing electron-dense material, were occasionally observed adjacent to stacks of cisternae of Golgi complexes. Groups of or individual small, round, oval or elongated dense granules were often seen. Polyribosomes

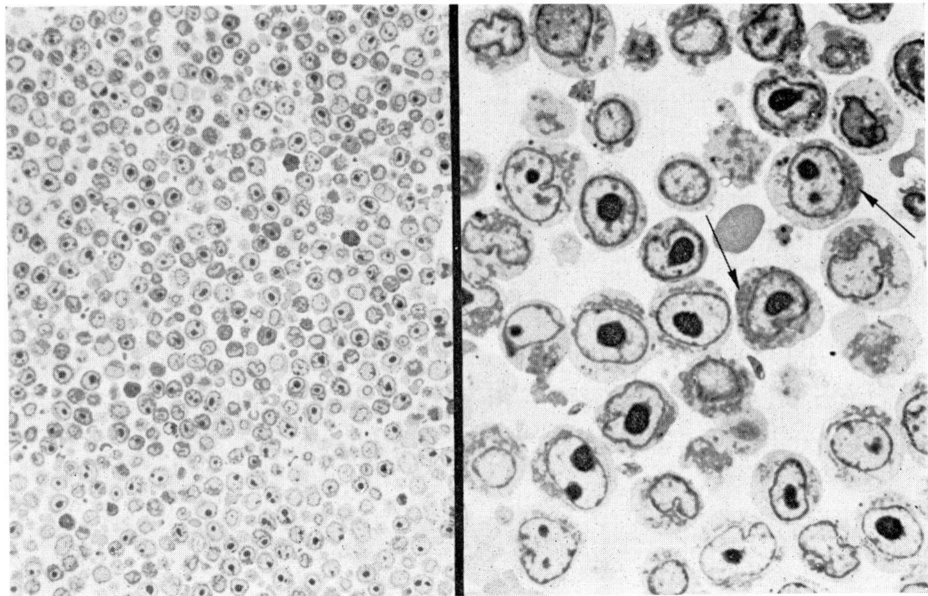

Figure 62. Epon-embedded, one-micron-thick section of leukemic cells from a patient with the leukemic phase of reticulum cell sarcoma. (*left*) The cells have large, fairly uniform nuclei, some of which are indented. These nuclei are vesicular and contain only small amounts of chromatin at the periphery. Most of the nuclei have a large, single, oval nucleolus while others have two smaller nucleoli (*right*). Within an area of the cytoplasm of some of the cells, small dense structures (arrows) which correspond to mitochondria can be seen.

and monoribosomes were scattered throughout the cytoplasm of all the leukemic cells, imparting the deep-blue color to the cytoplasm of cells stained with Wright's stain. Centrioles were seen in many cells, often associated with Golgi complexes (Fig. 63c). Membranes of rough endoplasmic reticulum were not plentiful but were seen scattered in the cytoplasm of all the leukemic cells.

In Plate 11 the leukemic cells from another patient with leukemic reticulum cell sarcoma are seen. These cells have pronounced monocytoid features characterized by multiple indentations in their nuclei and many chromatin aggregates. The cells obtained from the patient's bone marrow are similar (Plate 11).

Epon-embedded sections of leukemic cells from the peripheral blood of this patient showed some cells identical to those described above. In addition, leukemic cells with more pleomorphic, less vesicular nuclei containing smaller nucleoli were seen (Fig. 64). Electron microscopically, in addition to cells which were morphologically similar to those described in the first patient, leukemic cells from this patient with leukemic reticulum cell sarcoma had more ir-

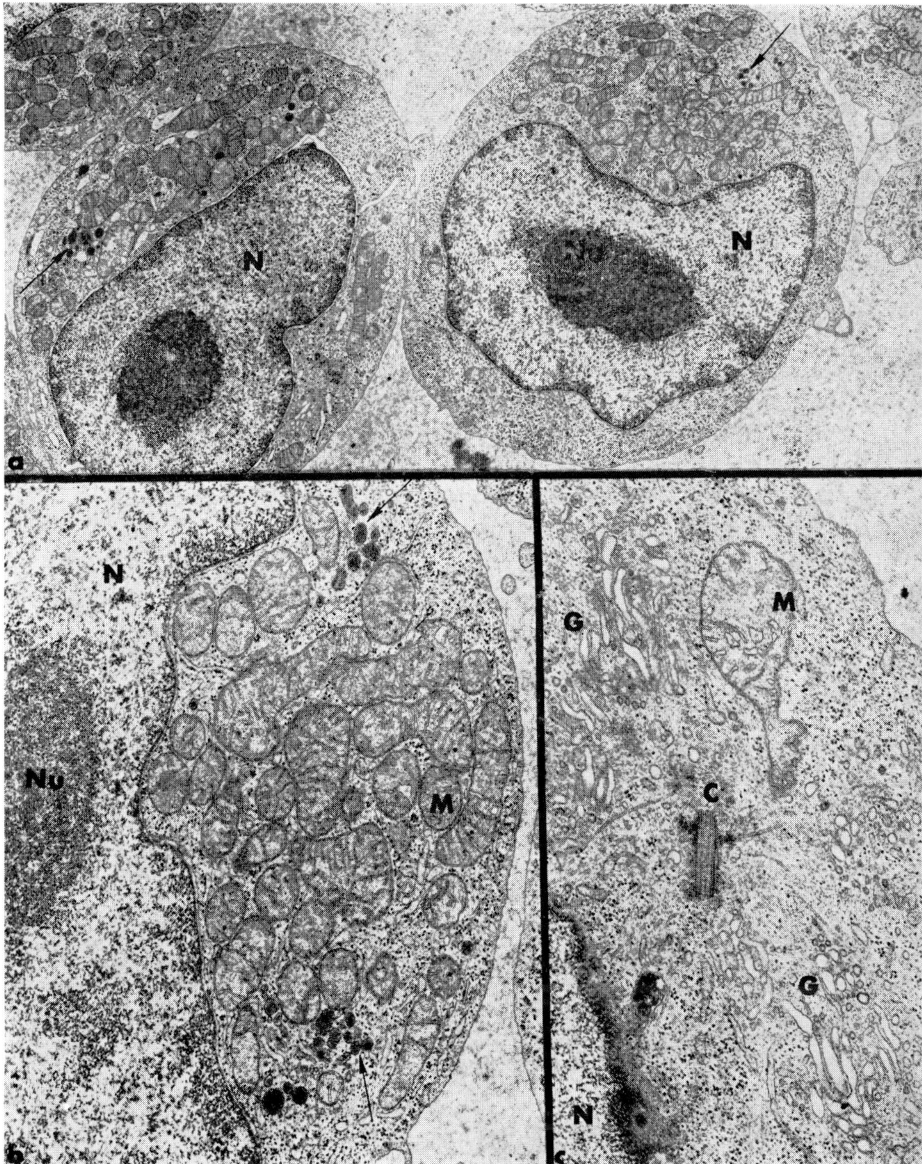

Figure 63. (a) Two leukemic cells from the peripheral blood of a patient with the leukemic phase of reticulum cell sarcoma. The nuclei (N) are irregular and contain mostly light-staining euchromatin and small amounts of granular clumped chromatin along the nuclear membrane. The nucleolus (Nu) in both cells is large and prominent. There is ample cytoplasm containing many mitochondria grouped in one part of the cell. Considerable variation in size and shape of these mitochondria is seen. There are many polyribosomes throughout the cytoplasm as well as occasional membranes of rough endoplasmic reticulum. Oval and elongated small, dense granules (arrows) are present at the periphery of the group of mitochondria. The cytoplasm contains numerous polyribosomes, monoribosomes and scattered membranes of rough endoplasmic reticulum. (c) A portion of a leukemic cell with well-developed Golgi complexes (G) surrounds a centriole (C). A large and irregularly shaped mitochondrion (M) is seen in the cytoplasm which contains numerous polyribosomes and occasional membranes of rough endoplasmic reticulum.

regular nuclei which contained more heterochromatin and smaller nucleoli (Fig. 65). These cells also had fewer mitochondria and less well developed Golgi complexes.

Ultrastructurally, the leukemic cells of reticulum cell sarcoma are readily differentiated from the cells of hairy cell leukemia (see ultrastructure of hairy cell leukemia).

Plate 12b and c shows the histiocytes observed in the peripheral blood of a third patient with reticulum cell sarcoma in the leukemic phase. These cells are large typical histiocytes with foamy vacuolated cytoplasm, pseudopodia and monocytoid nuclei. Cells obtained from the patient's marrow are seen in Plate 12a. They show marked monocytoid features, pseudopodia and cytoplasmic tails. The cells in this case are indistinguishable from leukemic cells in acute histiomonocytic leukemia.

Although some of the leukemic cells in leukemic reticulum cell sarcoma morphologically closely resemble cells described by Downey as being typical of leukemic reticuloendotheliosis, we prefer to use the more precise phrase "leukemic phase of reticulum cell sarcoma"

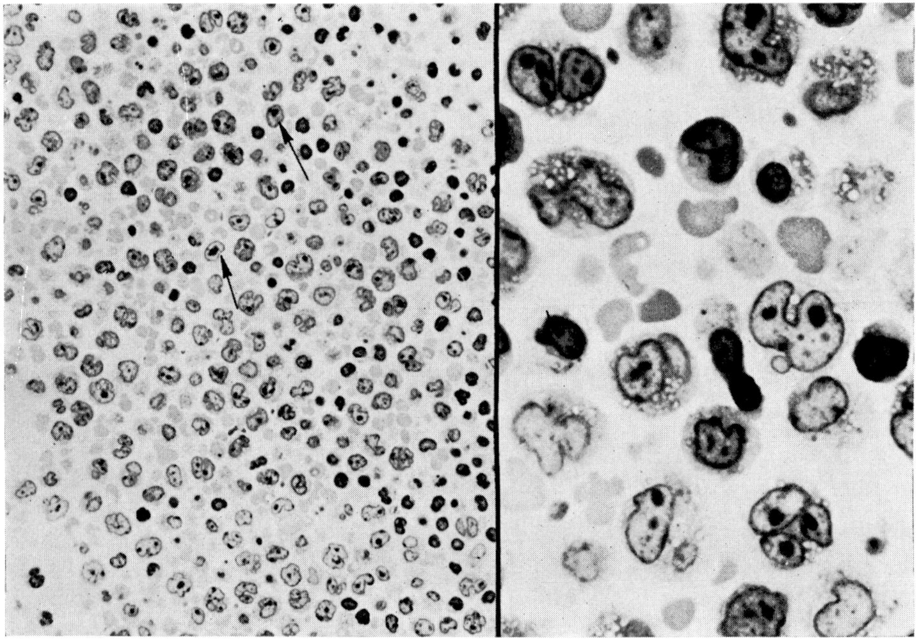

Figure 64. One-micron-thick section of leukemic cells from the peripheral blood of a patient with the leukemic phase of reticulum cell sarcoma. *(left)* Many of the cells have irregular nuclei with one or two nucleoli, while fewer cells have oval nuclei with a single, large and prominent nucleolus (arrows). *(right)* Higher magnification of the leukemic cells.

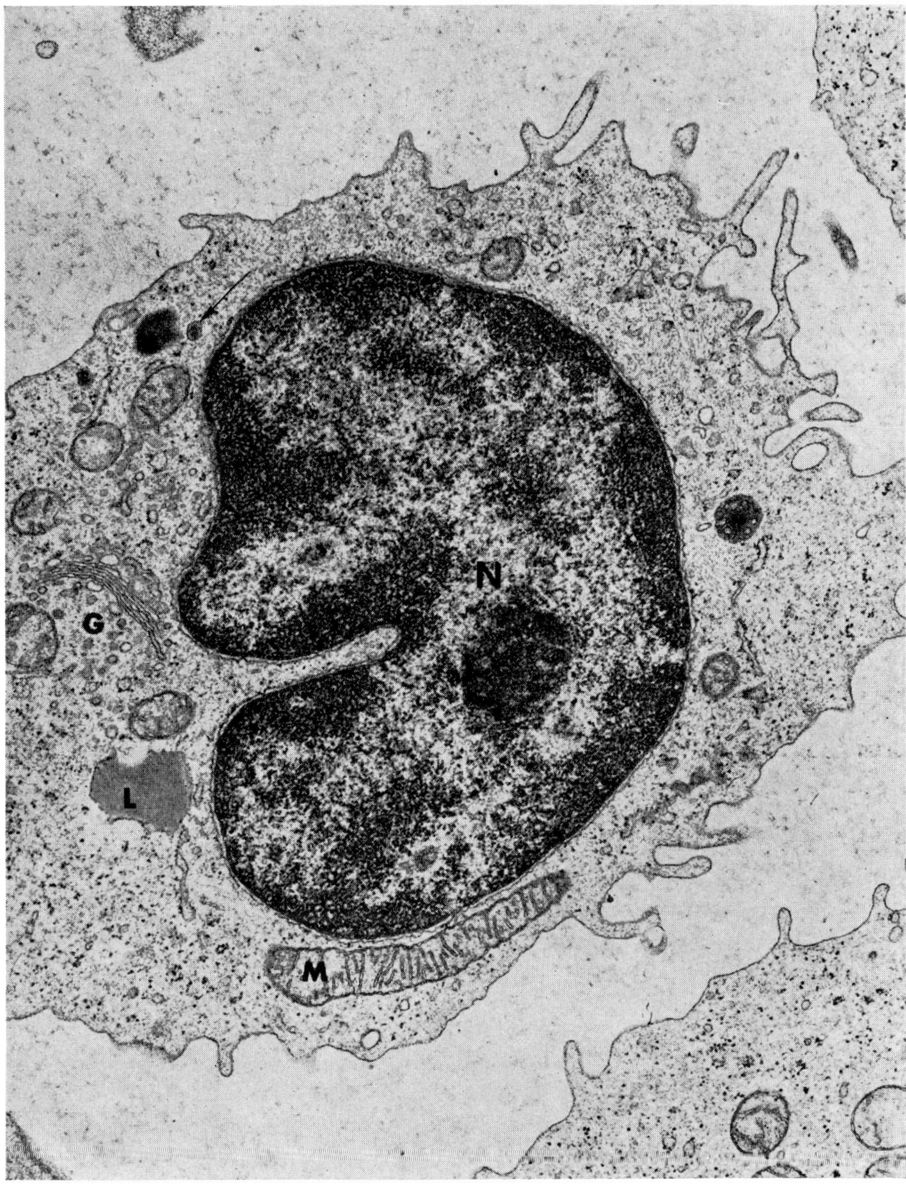

Figure 65. A leukemic cell from the peripheral blood of another patient with the leukemic phase of reticulum cell sarcoma. The indented nucleus (N) contains a considerable amount of heterochromatin and a prominent nucleolus. A moderate number of mitochondria (M) are seen in the cytoplasm. One mitochondrion has an elongated shape. Scattered monoribosomes, a few segments of rough endoplasmic reticulum, a Golgi complex (G), several granules (arrow) and a lipid body (L) are present in the cytoplasm.

for this type of leukemia, rather than the more ambiguous name "leukemic reticuloendotheliosis." The term "leukemic phase of reticulum cell sarcoma" indicates that this type of lymphoma has been diagnosed before the appearance of the leukemic phase.

Histiocytic Medullary Reticulosis

Another disorder which may be classified in the general but ambiguous category of reticuloses or neoplastic disorders of the reticuloendothelial system (217,229) is histiocytic medullary reticulosis. (29, 106,113,138,158,159,179,199,212,265,269,288,311) This disorder, which was described as a clinical and pathological entity in 1939 by Scott and Robb-Smith, (265) is characterized by lymphadenopathy, hepatosplenomegaly, fever, wasting, anemia, leukopenia and thrombocytopenia. The characteristic histiologic findings include a proliferation of malignant histiocytic cells including "prohistiocytes" (265) in lymph nodes, spleen, liver, bone marrow and sometimes the skin. Erythrophagocytosis by the histiocytic cells may be the cause of the anemia (217,302) and is often but not always a prominent feature of the disease. Although the patients are usually aleukemic, several reports describing a leukemic phase have appeared in the literature. (44,142) Rappaport (217) and Kingdon et al. (142) use the term "malignant histiocytosis" synonymously with "histiocytic medullary reticulosis," and they call the leukemic phase of malignant histiocytosis "histiocytic leukemia." The following terms, according to Rappaport, (217) are synonyms or variants of malignant histiocytosis: histiocytic leukemia, prohistiocytic medullary reticulosis, reticulum celled medullary reticulosis and reticulum cell leukemia.

Histologically, histiocytic medullary reticulosis or malignant histiocytosis must be differentiated from reticulum cell sarcoma (histiocytic lymphoma) in lymph node biopsies. In the former disorder, histiocytic cells are usually seen within the sinuses of the lymph node (Fig. 66) and are less cohesive than the neoplastic cells in reticulum cell sarcoma which also destroy the nodal architecure. When bizarre histiocytes and malignant giant cells are present, histiocytic medullary reticulosis may superficially simulate the morphological features of the reticular type of Hodgkin's disease.

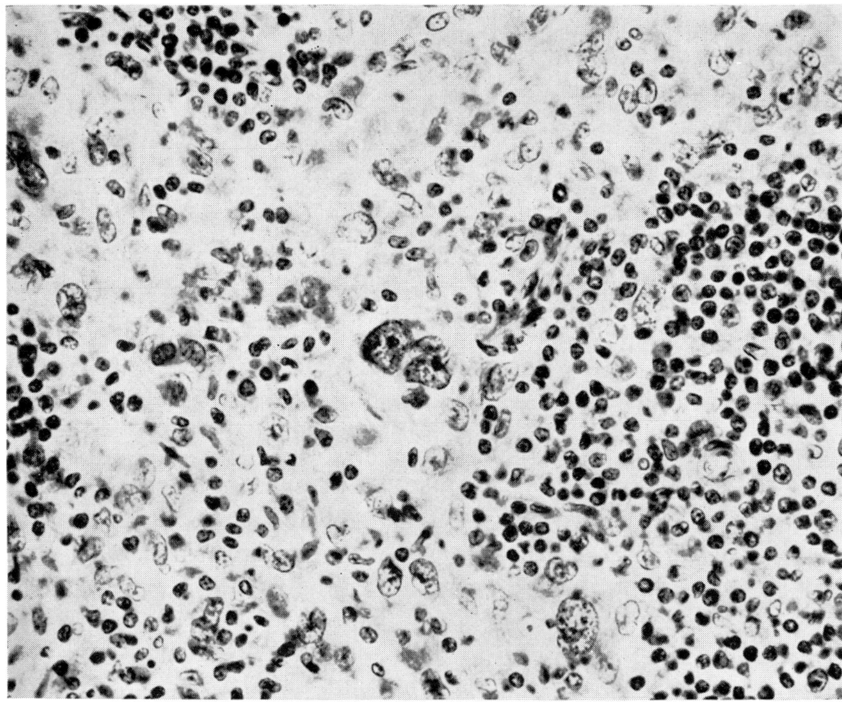

Figure 66. Lymph node biopsy from a patient with malignant histiocytosis (histiocytic medullary reticulosis). The widened sinusoid is filled with atypical and malignant histiocytic cells. A binucleate malignant histiocyte with large nucleoli resembling a Reed-Sternberg cell is seen.

CHAPTER VI

RELATIONSHIPS BETWEEN DISORDERS OF ERYTHROPOIESIS AND DISORDERS OF MONOCYTES

THE RELATIONSHIP BETWEEN DISORDERS of erythropoiesis and disorders of monocytes has been a topic of interest for some time (see Chapter II). Erythrophagocytosis by monocytes is a prominent feature of certain hemolytic anemias, (61) especially those characterized by elevated blood levels of cold agglutinins. In the latter conditions, the erythrocytes become coated with the IgM cold agglutinin. Specific receptor sites on the membrane of the monocyte show specificity for the immunoglobulin coating the red cell and along with the C^1 3 portion of complement (Chapter II), facilitate engulfment of the erythrocyte by the monocyte. This type of erythrophagocytosis by monocytes is illustrated in Figure 67a.

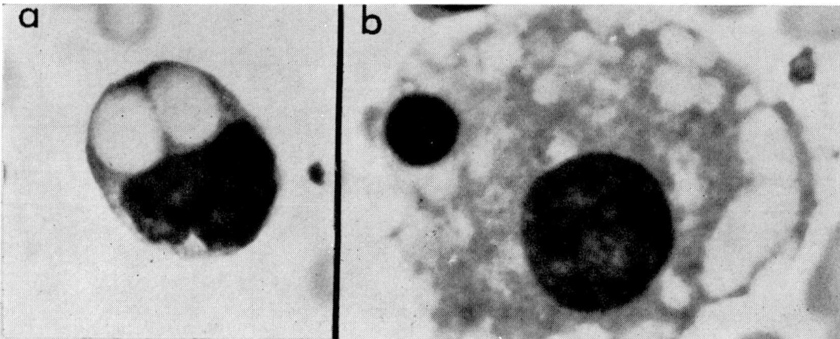

Figure 67. Erythrophagocytosis by mononuclear cells. (a) A monocyte which has ingested two mature erythrocytes in the peripheral blood of a patient with a high titer of cold agglutinins.

(b) Erythrophagocytosis of both mature erythrocytes and normoblasts (illustrated by the dark nucleus surrounded by rim of hemoglobinized cytoplasm) by a large neoplastic monocytoid reticulum cell in histiomonocytic leukemia.

The phenomenon of erythrophagocytosis by macrophages and histiocytes has been described in typhoid fever, (161) in subacute bacterial endocarditis (63,248,251) and in obscure anemias, (239,292) Erythrophagocytosis of immature erythrocytes by histiocytes is a common feature in the marrows of patients with the DiGuglielmo syndrome, and is the morphologic evidence for intramedullary red cell death (ineffective erythropoiesis) in this disease. (258)

Erythrophagocytosis may also occur in acute and subacute myeloblastic and myelomonocytic leukemia (Figs. 15,16d). Ackerman et al., (3) in a study of leukemic cells from a patient with "atypical myeloblastic leukemia," noted vacuoles containing mucopolysaccharide (presumably erythrocyte-derived) and erythrophagocytosis in some of the cells. Erythrophagocytosis of normoblasts and mature erythrocytes by monocytoid histiocytic cells is also seen in histiomonocytic leukemia (Fig. 67b) and in histiocytic medullary reticulosis.

A special relationship seems to exist between disorders of monocytes and the DiGuglielmo syndrome, also known as acute and chronic erythremic myelosis and erythroleukemia. DiGuglielmo (73) described acute erythremic myelosis as a disorder in which immature nucleated erythrocytes flooded the peripheral blood. DiGuglielmo (75) subsequently expanded his original findings and described blood and bone marrow findings in greater detail. Later, Dameshek and Baldini (68) and Dameshek (70) defined several diverse disorders of erythropoiesis including sideroachrestic anemia, (293) sideroblastic anemia, (8,24,60,124,125) acute and chronic erythremic myelosis, (73, 75) refractory anemia (20,32) and erythroleukemia (133,263,266) and grouped them under the general heading of DiGuglielmo syndrome.

DiGuglielmo syndrome is characterized by a refractory macrocytic anemia, (7) varying degrees of normoblastemia, splenomegaly and striking erythroid hyperplasia of the bone marrow. Proerythroblasts are increased in number, and the nuclear chromatin pattern of the intermediate normoblasts is usually megaloblastoid (see below). Because of the morphological abnormalities in granulocytes, megakaryocytes and erythroblasts, Dameshek (70) postulated that the DiGuglielmo syndrome was a panmyelosis and part of the myeloproliferative syndrome. Monocytosis is common in erythremic myelosis, (263) and DiGuglielmo himself (75) noted "monocytoid reticulum cells" in the marrows of many of his patients with the characteristic erythroid abnormalities.

Chromosomal aberrations, (67) deficiencies of heme synthetase and delta-Alase, (277) PAS positivity of the cytoplasm of proerythroblasts, (120) and electron microscopic evidence of abnormalities in the storage and transport of particulate iron (258) have been described in chronic erythremic myelosis. Cytochemical (139) abnormalities in the histones obtained from the nuclei of erythroid precursors in the DiGuglielmo syndrome have also been described.

The type of erythropoiesis in the DiGuglielmo syndrome has been called megaloblastoid by Heilmeyer and Schoener. (123) The distinguishing features of megaloblastoid erythropoiesis include block-like aggregates of chromatin connected to one another by thin chromatin strands, and an appreciable degree of fenestration of the nuclear chromatin. These nuclear features are generally seen in conjunction with nucleocytoplasmic asyncrony, particularly in macronormoblasts in which the cytoplasm appears to be more hemoglobinized than one would anticipate from the immaturity of the nuclear chromatin pattern. Typical megaloblastoid macronormoblasts are shown in Figure 68.

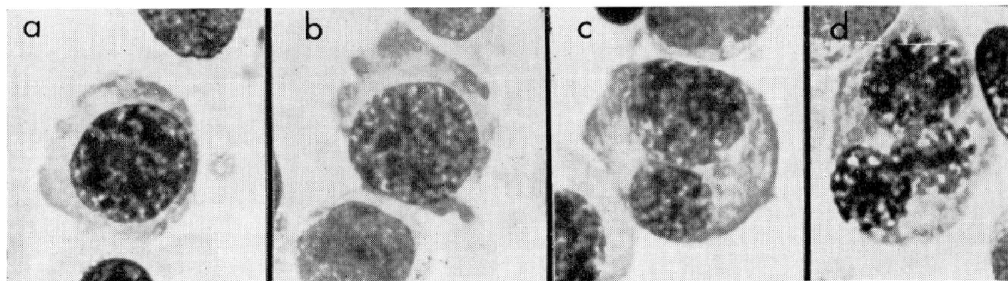

Figure 68. Erythroid abnormalities in myelomonocytic leukemia. (a) and (b) represent megaloblastoid intermediate macronormoblasts, (b) showing somewhat greater fenestration and attenuation of chromatin strands than (a).

(c) and (d) represent multinucleation and multiple lobulation of nuclei seen in erythroid precursors in this condition. The nuclear chromatin is megaloblastoid.

That megaloblastoid erythropoiesis may, in many instances, reflect an underlying neoplasia is suggested by the fact that a substantial number of patients with chronic erythremic myelosis subsequently develop acute leukemia, either myeloblastic, myelomonocytic or erythroleukemia. (69) Other authors have commented upon the relationship between disorders of erythropoiesis characterized by abnormal chromatin patterns in developing red cells and the subsequent development of acute leukemia. Vilter et al. (296) explored the relationship between refractory macrocytic anemia and monocytic leukemia. Vilter's type III refractory anemia with hyperplastic bone marrow and bizarre-appearing erythroid precursors frequently demonstrated evolution into acute "myelomonoblastic" leukemia. Type III refractory anemia may represent a preleukemic state as defined by Block et al., (26) and it has many features suggestive of the DiGuglielmo syndrome. Williams (303) described the development of acute myeloblastic leukemia (? myelomonocytic) following a prolonged period of refractory anemia, and Dubois-Ferriere et al. (81) described a case of marrow erythroblastosis accompanied by striking monocytosis in the peripheral blood. They noted that many of the monocytes appeared atypical and some showed erythrophagocytosis. Other cases in which disorders of erythropoiesis have either preceded or been coincident with neoplastic disorders of monocytes have been described by Block et al., (26) by Meacham and Weisberger (178) and by Broun (37) who called this combination "chronic erythromonocytic leukemia."

Figure 70 illustrates the bone marrow of a patient who was diagnosed as having chronic erythremic myelosis, as defined by Dameshek. (70) The hyperplasia of proerythroblasts with a "maturation arrest" at this level of development along with the increased numbers of megaloblastoid intermediate macronormoblasts is apparent (Fig. 69a). Several months after the diagnosis of chronic erythremic myelosis was made, large numbers of neoplastic monocytes appeared in the peripheral blood, and the bone marrow showed acute myelomonocytic leukemia (Fig. 69b).

Reasons why refractory macrocytic anemias of the DiGuglielmo type are so frequently precursors or forerunners of acute or subacute myelomonocytic leukemia remain speculative. It has been well established, however, that in many of these refractory anemias, usually of the DiGuglielmo variety, chromosomal aberrations including deletions and translocations (70) are common. These abnormalities imply that the refractory anemia itself, and particularly the erythroid precursors involved, are neoplastic *de novo*. Why a myeloblastic or myelomonocytic leukemia in particular rather than another cytological type should evolve from this anemia is not yet understood.

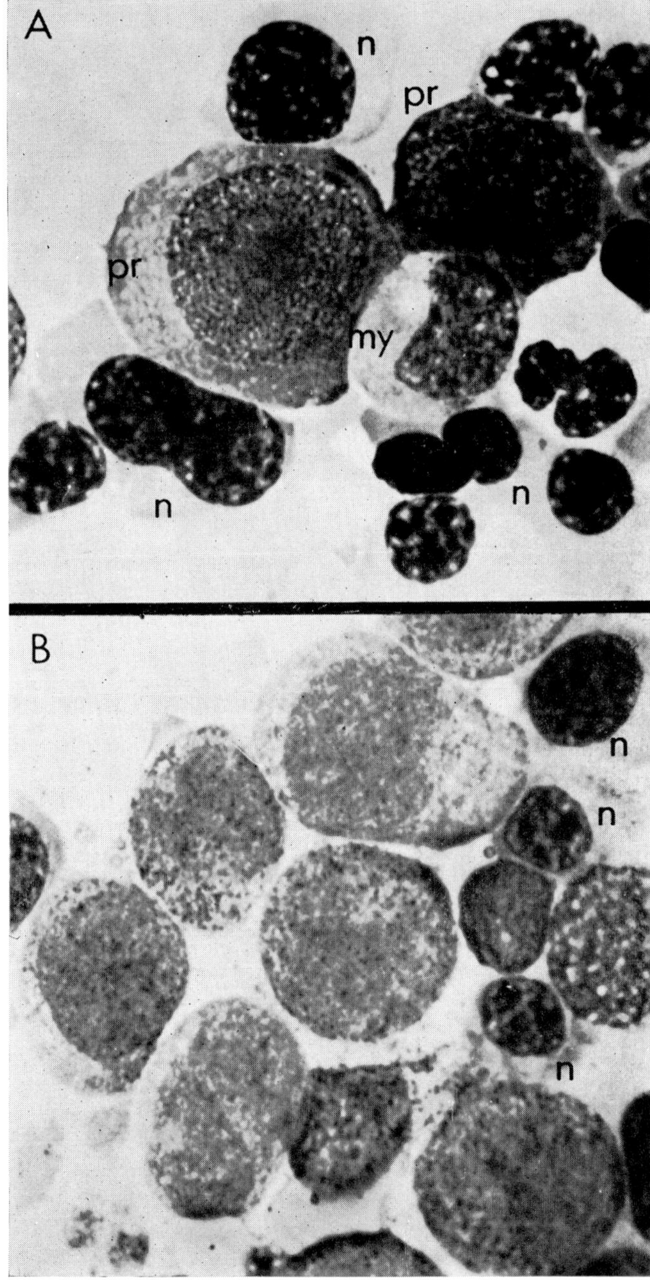

Figure 69. (A) Cells from the bone marrow of a patient with chronic erythremic myelosis. Large proerythroblasts (pr) along with aberrant-appearing megaloblastoid intermediate macronormoblasts (n) and a myelocyte (my) can be seen.

(B) Approximately two months after the diagnosis of erythremic myelosis was made
in this patient, his bone marrow revealed acute myelomonocytic leukemia, as can be
seen in this photomicrograph. Numerous monocytoid blasts with adundant cytoplasmic
granules are seen, as well as several megaloblastoid intermediate macronormoblasts (n).

BIBLIOGRAPHY

1. Abramson, N.; Gelfand, E. W.; Jandl, J. H. and Rosen, F. S.: The interaction between human monocytes and red cells. Specificity for IgG subclasses and IgG fragments. *J Exp Med, 132:* 1207, 1970.

2. ———; LoBuglio, A. F.; Jandl, J. H. and Cotran, R. S.: The interaction between human monocytes and red cells. Binding characteristics. *J Exp Med, 132:* 1191, 1970.

3. Ackerman, G. A.; Grasso, J. A. and Knouff, R. A.: Morphological and histiochemical studies of the leukemic cells from a patient with atypical myeloblastic leukemia with special reference to intracytoplasmic mucopolysaccharide vacuoles and fibrillar formation. *Blood, 16:* 1253, 1960.

4. Anderson, D. R.: Ultrastructure of normal and leukemic leukocytes in human peripheral blood. *J Ultrastruct Res (Suppl), 9:* 5, 1966.

5. Asamer, H.; Schmalzl, F. and Braunsteiner, H.: The immunocytologic determination of lysozyme in human blood cells. *Acta Haematol, 41:* 49, 1969.

6. Bakalos, D.: *Monocytic Precursors and Their Significance. Atlas of Bone Marrow and Lymph Node Cytology.* Athens, G. Parissianos, 1965.

7. Baldini, M.; Fudenberg, H. H.; Fukatake, K. and Dameshek, W.: The anemia of the DiGuglielmo syndrome. *Blood, 14:* 334, 1959.

8. Barry, W. E. and Day, H. J.: Refractory sideroblastic anemia. Clinical and hematologic study of ten cases. *Ann Intern Med, 61:* 1029, 1964.

9. Beattie, J. W.; Seal, R. M. E. and Crowther, K. V.: Chronic monocytic leukemia. *Q J Med, 78:* 131, 1957.

10. Belding, L.; Daland, B. A. and Parker, F., Jr.: Histiocytic and monocytic leukemia. A clinical, hematologic, and pathological differentiation. *Cancer, 8:* 237, 1955.

11. Bennett, J. M.: Myelomonocytic leukemia: A historical review and perspective. *Cancer, 27:* 1218, 1971.

12. Bennett, W. E. and Cohn, Z. A.: The isolation and selected properties of blood monocytes. *J Exp Med, 123:* 145, 1966.

13. Berg, B. and Bradt, R.: The cytology, distribution, and function of the neoplastic cells in leukaemic reticuloendotheliosis. *Scand J Haematol, 7:* 428, 1970.

14. Berkheiser, S. W.: Studies on the comparative morphology of monocytic leukemia, granulocytic leukemia, and reticulum cell sarcoma. *Cancer, 10:* 606, 1957.

15. Bessis, M.: *Cytology of the Blood and Blood-Forming Organs.* New York, Grune and Stratton, 1956.

16. ——— and Breton-Gorius, J.: Examen au microscope électronique des cellules des leucémies myeloides. *Bull Mic Appl, 5:* 9, 1957.

17. ——— and Thiery, J. P.: Electron microscopy of human white blood cells and their stem cells. *Int Rev Cytol, 12:* 199, 1961.

18. ——— and Jensen, W. N.: Sideroblastic anaemia, mitochondria and erythroblastic iron. *Br J Haematol, 11:* 49, 1965.

19. ———: Ultrastructure of normal and leukemic granulocytes. In C. J. D. Zarafonetis (Ed.): *Proceedings of the International Conference on Leukemia-Lymphoma.* Philadelphia, Lea and Febiger, p. 281, 1968.

20. ———; Dreyfus, B.; Breton-Gorius, J. and Sultan, C.: Etude au microscope électronique des onze cas d'anemies réfractaires avec enzymopathies multiples. *Nouv Rev Fr Hematol, 9:* 87, 1969.

21. ——— and Breton-Gorius, J.: Pathologie et asynchronisme du development des

organelles cellulatres au cours des leucémies aigues granulocytaires. *Nouv Rev Fr Hematol, 9:* 245, 1969.

22. Bianchi, L.: Richerche sperimentali ed istopathologiche sull'infezione da Bacterium Monocytogenes nel coniglio. *Hematol, 11:* 163, 1930.

23. Bingel, P.: Monozytenleukaemie. *Deutsch Med Wochenschr, 42:* 1503, 1916.

24. Bjorkman, S. E.: Chronic refractory anemia with sideroblastic bone marrow. A study of four cases. *Blood, 2:* 250, 1956.

25. Blair, T. R.; Bayrd, E. D. and Pease, G. L.: Atypical leukemia. *JAMA, 198:* 21, 1966.

26. Block, M.; Jacobson, L. O. and Bethard, W. F.: Preleukemic acute human leukemia. *JAMA, 152:* 1018, 1953.

27. Bloom, W.: The origin and nature of the monocyte. *Folia Haematol, 37:* 1, 1928.

28. ———: The relationships between lymphocytes, monocytes and plasma cells. *Folia Haematol, 37:* 63, 1928.

29. Boake, W. C.; Card, W. H. and Kimmey, J. F.: Histiocytic medullary reticulosis: Concurrence in father and son. *Arch Intern Med, 116:* 245, 1965.

30. Bock, H. E. and Wiede, K.: Zur Frage der leukaemischen Reticuloendotheliosen (Monocytenleukaemie). *Virchows Arch, 276:* 553, 1930.

31. Bodel, P. and Athius, E.: Release of endogenous pyrogen by human monocytes. *N Engl J Med, 276:* 1002, 1967.

32. Boniford, R. P. and Rhoads, C. P.: Refractory anemia. I. Clinical and pathological aspects. *Q J Med, 10:* 175, 1941.

33. Bornstein, R. S.; Theologides, A. and Kennedy, B. J.: Daunorubricine in acute myelogenous leukemia in adults. *JAMA, 207:* 1301, 1969.

34. Bouroncle, B. A.; Wiseman, B. K. and Doan, C. A.: Leukemic reticuloendotheliosis. *Blood, 13:* 609, 1958.

35. Brenton-Gorius, T. and Guichard, T.: Etude au microscope électronique de la localisation des peroxidases dans les cellules de la moelle osseuse humaine. *Nouv Rev Fr Hematol, 9:* 678, 1969.

36. Brody, J. I.; Cypress, E.; Kimball, S. and McKenzie, D.: The Sézary syndrome. A unique cutaneous reticulosis. *Arch Intern Med, 110:* 205, 1962.

37. Broun, G. O.: Chronic erythromonocytic leukemia. *Am J Med, 47:* 785, 1969.

38. Brucher, H.: The monocytes. In H. Braunsteiner and D. Zucker-Franklin (Eds.): *The Physiology and Pathology of Leukocytes.* New York, Grune and Stratton, p. 91, 1962.

39. Bunting, C. H.: The blood picture in Hodgkin's disease. *Johns Hopkins Hosp Bull, 25:* 173, 1914.

40. Bykowa, O.: Die Reaktion des reticulo-endothelialen Systems und die septische Infektion. *Folia Haematol, 48:* 408, 1932.

41. Capone, R. J.; Weinreb, E. L. and Chapman, G. B.: Electron microscope studies on normal human myeloid elements. *Blood, 23:* 300, 1964.

42. Cattaneo, L.: Contributo allo studio della genesi dei monociti. *Haematol, 12:* 568, 1931.

43. Citron, J.: Ueber zwei bemerkenswerte Faelle von (akuter) Leukaemie. *Folia Haematol, 20:* 1, 1915.

44. Clark, B. S. and Dawson, P. J.: Histiocytic medullary reticulosis presenting with a leukemic blood picture. *Am J Med, 47:* 314, 1969.

45. Clark, E. R. and Clark, E. L.: Relation of monocytes of the blood to the tissue macrophages. *Am J Anat, 46:* 149, 1930.

46. Cline, M. J. and Lehrer, R. I.: Phagocytosis by human monocytes. *Blood, 32:* 423, 1968.

47. ———— and Swett, V. C.: The interaction of human monocytes and lymphocytes. *J Exp Med, 128:* 1309, 1968.

48. Clough, P. W.: Monocytic leukemia. *Assn Am Phys (Tr), 46:* 258, 1931.

49. ————: Monocytic leukemia. *Bull Johns Hopkins Hosp, 51:* 148, 1932.

50. Cohn, Z. A.: The fate of bacteria within phagocytic cells. I. The degradation of isotopically labeled bacteria by polymorphonuclear leucocytes and macrophages. *J Exp Med, 117:* 27, 1963.

51. ———— and Benson, B.: The differentiation of mononuclear phagocytes: Morphology, cytochemistry, and biochemistry. *J Exp Med, 121:* 153, 1965.

52. ———— and Benson, B.: The *in vitro* differentiation of mononuclear phagocytes. I. The influence of inhibitors and the results of autoradiography. *J Exp Med, 121:* 279, 1965.

53. ————; Hirsh, J. G. and Fedorko, M. E.: The *in vitro* differentiation of mono-phagocytes. IV. The ultra-structure of macrophage differentiation in the peritoneal cavity and in culture. *J Exp Med, 123:* 757, 1966.

54. ————: The structure and function of monocytes and macrophages. *In* F. J. Dixon and H. G. Kempel (Eds.): *Advances in Immunology.* New York, Academic Press, vol. 9, p. 163, 1968.

55. Cole, J. P.: The Significance of Phagocytic Reticuloendothelial Cell in Blood Smears from the Ear in Patients with Subacute Bacterial Endocarditis. Thesis. Graduate School, University of Minnesota, 1951.

56. Cooke, W. E.: Acute monocytic (histiocytic) leukemia. *Lancet, 221:* 129, 1931.

57. Crowther, D.; Bateman, C. J. R.; Vartan, C. P.; Whitehouse, J. M. A.; Malpas, J. S.; Fairley, G. H. and Scott, R. B.: Combination chemotherapy using l-asparaginase, daunorubicin and cytosine arabinoside in adults with acute myelogenous leukemia. *Br Med J, 4:* 513, 1970.

58. Cunningham, R. S.; Sabin, F. R. and Doan, C. A.: The development of leukocytes, lymphocytes and monocytes from a specific stem cell in adult tissue. *Carnegie Contrib Embryol, 16:* 227, 1925.

59. ———— and Tompkins, E. H.: The supravital staining of normal human blood cells. *Folia Haematol, 42:* 257, 1930.

60. Dacie, J. V.; Smith, M. D.; White, J. C. and Mollin, D. L.: Refractory normoblastic anaemia: a clinical and haematological study of seven cases. *Br J Haematol, 5:* 56, 1959.

61. ————: *The Haemolytic Anaemias.* New York, Grune and Stratton, 1960.

62. ———— and Mollin, D. L.: Siderocytes, sideroblasts and sideroblastic anaemia. *Acta Med Scand (Suppl), 445:* 237, 1966.

63. Daland, G. A.; Gottlieb, L.; Wallerstein, R. O. and Castle, W. B.: Hematologic observations in bacterial endocarditis: especially the prevalence of histiocytes and the elevation and variation of the white cell count in blood from the ear lobe. *J Lab Clin Med, 48:* 827, 1956.

64. Dalrymple-Champney, W.: Undulant fever: a neglected problem. *Lancet, 1:* 477, 1950.

65. Dameshek, W.: Acute monocytic (histiocytic) leukemia. *Arch Intern Med, 46:* 718, 1930.

66. ————: The appearance of histiocytes in the peripheral blood. *Arch Intern Med, 47:* 968, 1931.

67. ——: Proliferative disease of the reticuloendothelial system. II. Aleukemic reticulosis. *Folia Haematol, 49:* 64, 1933.

68. —— and Baldini, M.: The DiGuglielmo syndrome. *Blood, 13:* 192, 1958.

69. —— and Gunz, F.: *Leukemia.* 2nd ed. New York, Grune and Stratton, 1964.

70. ——: Sideroblastic anemia. Is this a malignancy? *Br J Haematol, 11:* 52, 1965.

71. Darr, A. D. and Moloney, W. C.: Acquired pseudo-Pelger Huet anomaly of granulocytic leukocytes. *N Engl J Med, 261:* 742, 1959.

72. dePetris, S.; Karlsbad, G. and Pernis, B.: Filamentous structures in the cytoplasm of normal mononuclear phagocytes. *J Ultrastruct Res, 7:* 39, 1962.

73. DiGuglielmo, G.: Le eritremie. *Haematol, 9:* 301, 1928.

74. ——; Morrelli, A. and Maurea, C.: Istioleucemica chronica. *Haematol, 37:* 1, 1933.

75. ——: Les maladies érythremiques. *Rev Hematol, 1:* 355, 1946.

76. Doan, C. A. and Wiseman, B. K.: The monocytes, monocytosis, and monocytic leukosis: a clinical and pathological study. *Ann Intern Med, 8:* 383, 1934.

77. Downey, H.: Origin of monocytes in monocytic leukemia and leukemic reticuloendotheliosis. *Anat Rec, 48:* 16, 1931.

78. ——: The myeloblast. In E. V. Cowdrey: *Special Cytology.* New York, P. B. Hoeber, vol. 1, p. 371, 1932.

79. ——: Monocytic leucemia and leucemic reticuloendotheliosis. In H. Downey: *Handbook of Hematology.* New York, P. H. Hoeber, vol. 9, p. 1275, 1938.

80. ——: The myeloblast. In H. Downey: *Handbook of Hematology.* New York, P. B. Hoeber, p. 1963, 1938.

81. DuBois-Ferriere, H.; Chapius-Hoffmann, J.; Hurni, A. and Cruchaud, A.: Erythroblastomatose diffuse avec reaction monocytaire sanguine. *Schweitz Med Wochnschr, 85:* 946, 1955.

82. Ebert, R. H. and Florey, H. W.: The extravascular development of the monocyte observed in vivo. *Br J Exp Pathol, 20:* 347, 1939.

83. Ehrenrich, B. A. and Cohen, Z. A.: Pinocytosis by macrophages. *J Reticuloendothel Soc, 5:* 230, 1968.

84. Ehrlich, P.: Ueber die spezifischen Granulationen des Blutes. *Arch Anat Physiol Phys Abth,* p. 571, 1879.

85. ——: Methodologische Beiträge zur Physiologie und Pathologie der verschiedenen Formen der Leukocyten. *Z Klin Med, 1:* 553, 1880.

86. —— and Lazarus, A.: Histology of the blood. Normal and pathological. In H. Nothnagel: *Diseases of the Blood.* New York, W. B. Saunders, 1905, p. 17.

87. Eliot, C.: The origin of the phagocytic cells in the rabbit. *Johns Hopkins Hosp Bull, 39:* 149, 1926.

88. Ellison, R. R. and Holland, J. F.: Arabinosyl cytosine, a useful agent in the treatment of acute leukemia in adults. *Blood, 32:* 507, 1968.

89. Evans, T. S.: Monocytic leukemia. *Medicine, 21:* 421, 1942.

90. Ewald, O.: Die leukaemische Retikuloendotheliose. *Deutsch Arch Klin Med, 142:* 222, 1923.

91. Ewing, J.: Endothelioma of lymph nodes. *J Med Res, 28:* 1, 1913.

92. Fedorko, M. E. and Hirsch, J. G.: Structure of monocytes and macrophages. *Sem Hematol, 7:* 109, 1970.

93. Ferrata, A.: Studi sulle emopatie. I. Sulla istogenesi della leucemia granulocitica. *Haematol, 2:* 242, 1921.

94. ———: Studi sulle emopatie. II. Ancora sull'istogenesi della leucemia granulo-citica. *Haematol, 5:* 228, 1924.

95. Fleischmann, P.: Der zweite Fall von Monozyten-leukaemie. *Folia Haematol, 20:* 17, 1915.

96. Foord, A. G.; Parsons, L. and Butt, E. M.: Leukemic reticuloendotheliosis (mono-cytic leukemia). *JAMA, 101:* 1859, 1933.

97. Forkner, C. E.: Material from lymph nodes. IV. The heterology of lymphoid tissue with special reference to the monocyte supravital studies. *J Exp Med, 49:* 323, 1929.

98. ———: The origin of monocytes in certain lymph nodes and their genetic relations to other connective tissue cells. *J Exp Med, 52:* 385, 1930.

99. ———: Clinical and pathological differentiation of acute leukemia with special reference to acute monocytic leukemia. *Arch Intern Med, 53:* 1, 1934.

100. Fowler, W. M.: Monocytic leucemia. *J Lab Clin Med, 18:* 1260, 1932.

101. Franco, E. E.: Contribuzione alla conoscenza dell' anatomia patologica della leishmanosi cutanio-mucosa od americana. *Arch Sci Med, 43:* 246, 1920.

102. Freeman, A. I. and Journey, L. F.: Ultrastructural studies on monocytic leukemia. *Br J Haematol, 20:* 225, 1971.

103. Freeman, H. E. and Koletsky, S.: Cutaneous lesions in monocytic leukemia. Report of two cases with pathologic study. *Arch Dermatol, 40:* 218, 1939.

104. Freeman, J. A. and Samuels, M. S.: The ultrastructure of a fibrillar formation of leukaemic human blood. *Blood, 13:* 725, 1958.

105. Friereich, F. J.; Bodey, G. R.; Hart, J. S.; Whitecar, J. P.; McCredie, J. R. and McCredie, K. B.: Current status of therapy for adult leukemia. *Recent Results Cancer Res, 36:* 119, 1971.

106. Friedman, R. M. and Steigbigel, N. H.: Histiocytic medullary reticulosis. *Am J Med, 38:* 130, 1965.

107. Garvin, R. D. and Bargen, J. A.: The hematologic picture of chronic ulcerative colitis: its relation to prognosis and treatment. *Am J Med Sci, 193:* 744, 1937.

108. Gee, T. S.; Hu, K. P. and Clarkson, B. D.: Treatment of adult acute leukemia with arabinosyl cytosine and thioguanine. *Cancer, 23:* 1019, 1969.

109. Ghadially, F. N. and Skinnider, L. F.: Ultrastructure of hairy cell leukemia. *Cancer, 29:* 444, 1972.

110. Gibson, A.: Monocytic leukaemoid reaction associated with tuberculosis and mediastinal teratoma. *J Pathol Bacteriol, 58:* 469, 1946.

111. Gohn, A. and Roman, B.: Ueber das Lymphosarcom. *Frank. Z Pathol, 19:* 1, 1916.

112. Goormaghtigh, N.: Malignant proliferation of reticuloendothelial tissue of lym-phatic glands. *Compte Soc Biol, 92:* 457, 1925.

113. Greenberg, E.; Cohen, D. M.; Pease, L. and Kyle, R. A.: Histiocytic medullary reticulosis. *Proc Stf Mtg Mayo Clinic, 37:* 271, 1962.

114. Greenburg, P. L.; Nichols, W. C. and Schrier, S. L.: Granulopoiesis in acute myeloid leukemia and preleukemia. *N Engl J Med, 284:* 1225, 1971.

115. Haffley, G. N. and Schipfer, L. A.: Subacute monocytic leukemia with nasal manifestations. *Arch Otolaryngol, 31:* 858, 1940.

116. Hall, B. E.: A critical review of the hematological literature dealing with the results of the supranatal staining method. *Folia Haematol, 43:* 206, 1930.

117. Hanifin, J. M. and Cline, M. J.: Human monocytes and macrophages. Interaction with antigen and lymphocytes. *J Cell Biol, 46:* 97, 1970.

118. Hawksley, J. C.: A note on the occurrence of Auer bodies in monocytic leukaemia. *J Pathol Bacteriol, 40:* 365, 1938.

119. Hayhoe, F. G. J.: *Leukaemia. Research and Clinical Practice.* Boston, Little, Brown and Co., 1960.

120. ———; Guaglino, D. and Doll, R.: The cytology and cytochemistry of acute leukaemias. In *M. R. C. Special Reports Series, No. 304.* H. M. Stationery Office, London. 1964.

121. ——— and Cawley, J. C.: Acute leukaemia: cellular morphology, cytochemistry, and fine structure. *Clinics in Haematol, 1:* 49, 1972.

122. Heckner, F.: *Leitfaden der Blutzellkunde.* Munchen u. Berlin, Urben u. Schwarzenberg Verlag, 1965.

123. Heilmeyer, L. and Schoener, W.: Die chronische Erythroblastose des Erwachsenen als leukaemie-paralleler Prozess des erythrocytaeren Systems. *Deutsch Arch Klin Med, 187:* 223, 1941.

124. ———; Keiderling, W.; Bilger, R. and Bernauer, H.: Ueber chronische refraktaere Anaemie mit sideroblastischem Knochenmark (anaemia refractria sideroblastica). *Folia Haematol (Frankfurt), 2:* 49, 1958.

125. ———: *Disturbances in Heme Synthesis.* Springfield, Thomas, 1966.

126. Hickling, R. A.: The monocytes in pneumonia. *Arch Intern Med, 40:* 594, 1927.

127. Hill, R. W. and Bayrd, E. D.: Phagocytic reticuloendothelial cells in subacute bacterial endocarditis with negative cultures. *Ann Intern Med, 52:* 310, 1960.

128. Hirsch, J. G. and Fedorko, M. E.: Ultrastructure of human leukocytes after simultaneous fixation with glutaraldehyde and osmium tetroxide and "postfixation" in uranyl acetate. *J Cell Biol, 38:* 615, 1968.

129. Huber, H.; Polley, N. M.; Linscott, W. D.; Fudenberg, H. H. and Muller-Eberhard, H. J.: Human monocytes: distinct receptor sites for the third component of complement and for immunoglobulin G. *Science, 126:* 128, 1968.

130. Hurxthal, L. M.: Clinical observations in subacute bacterial endocarditis. *Boston Med J, 197:* 41, 1927.

131. Isaacs, R. and Sturgis, C. C.: Types of monocytic leukemia. *Ann Am Phys Trans, 51:* 40, 1936.

132. ———: Lymphosarcoma cell leukemia. *Ann Intern Med, 11:* 657, 1937.

133. Israels, M. C. G.: Immature cell erythraemia in an adult. *J Pathol Bacteriol, 48:* 299, 1939.

134. Jacobsen, K. M.: Monozytenleukose. *Acta Med Scand, 30:* 205, 1942.

135. Jaffe, R. H.: Morphology of the inflammatory defense reactions in leukemia. *Arch Pathol, 14:* 177, 1932.

136. ———: The reticuloendothelial system. In H. Downey (Ed.): *Handbook of Hematology.* New York, Hoeber, 1938, p. 971.

137. Kakefuda, T.: Electron microscopy of normal and leukemic cells. In G. D. Amromin: *Pathology of Leukemia.* New York, P. B. Hoeber, 1968.

138. Kamegaya, K. and Noguchi, H.: Histiocytic medullary reticulosis (reticuloendotheliosis with striking erythrophagocytosis). *Acta Pathol Jap, 14:* 231, 1964.

139. Kass, L.: Demonstration of histones in proerythroblasts in pernicious anemia and the DiGuglielmo syndrome. *J Histochem Cytochem, 20:* 817, 1972.

140. ———: *Bone Marrow Interpretation.* Springfield, Thomas, 1973.

141. Katayama, I.; Li, C. Y. and Ham, L. T.: Ultrastructural characteristics of the 'hairy cells' of leukemic reticuloendotheliosis. *Am J Pathol, 67:* 361, 1972.

142. Kingdon, H. S.; Baron, J. M.; Byrne, G. E. and Rappaport, H.: Malignant histio-

cytosis. Results of combination vincristine-prednisone therapy. *Ann Intern Med, 72:* 705, 1970.

143. Leder, L. D. and Nicolas, R.: Fermentcytochemische Untersuchungen zur Genese der Macrophagen an Hautfenster Preparaeten. *Frankfurt Z Pathol, 73:* 228, 1963.

144. ————: Ueber die selektive fermentcytochemische Darstellung von neutrophilen myeloischen Zellen und Gewebsmastzellen im Paraffinschmitt. *Klin Kochenschr, 42:* 553, 1964.

145. ————: The origin of blood monocytes and macrophages. *Blut, 16:* 86, 1967.

146. ————: Der Herkunft der Blutmonozyten und ihre Beziehungen zu den sog. Histiozyten. In *Der Monozyt. Deutsche Gesellschaft fur Haematologie.* Munich, J. F. Lehmanns Verlag, 1969.

147. Lee, S. L.; Rosner, F. and Rosenthal, R. L.: Reticulum cell leukemia. Clinical and hematologic entity. *N Y J Med, 69:* 422, 1969.

148. Leir, J. A.; Vincent, P. C. and Gunz, F. W.: Combination chemotherapy of adult acute non-lymphoblastic leukemia. *Ann Intern Med, 76:* 397, 1972.

149. Levine, V.: Monocytic leukemia: report of nine cases. *Folia Haematol, 52:* 305, 1934.

150. Levinson, B.; Walter, B. A.; Wintrobe, M. M. and Cartwright, G. E.: A clinical study of Hodgkin's disease. *Arch Intern Med, 99:* 519, 1957.

151. Lewis, M. R. and Lewis, W. H.: Transformation of mononuclear blood-cells into macrophages, epithelioid cells, and giant cells in hanging-drop blood cultures from lower vertebrates. *Carneg Cont Enb, 18:* 95, 1925.

152. Linman, J. W.: Myelomonocytic leukemia and its preleukemic phase. *J Chronic Dis, 22:* 713, 1970.

153. Lipson, R. L.; Bayrd, E. D. and Watkins, C. H.: The postsplenectomy blood picture. *Am J Clin Pathol, 32:* 526, 1959.

154. LoBuglio, A. F.; Cotran, R. S. and Jandl, J. H.: Red cells coated with immunoglobulin G: binding and sphering by mononuclear cells in man. *Science, 158:* 1582, 1967.

155. Low, F. and Freeman, J.: *Electron Microscopic Atlas of Normal and Leukemic Human Blood.* New York, McGraw-Hill, 1958.

156. Lowenbraun, S.; Sutherland, J. C.; Feldman, M. J. and Serpick, A. A.: Transformation of reticulum cell sarcoma to acute leukemia. *Cancer, 27:* 579, 1971.

157. Lukes, R. J.: The pathological picture of the malignant lymphomas. In C. J. D. Zarafonetis (Ed.): *Proceedings of the International Conference on Leukemia-Lymphoma.* Philadelphia, Lea and Febiger, 1968, p. 331.

158. Lutman, G. B. and Senhauser, D. A.: Histiocytic medullary reticulosis: report of a case with autopsy findings. *South Med, 59:* 1345, 1966.

159. Lynch, E. C. and Alfred, C. P.: Histiocytic medullary reticulosis. Hemolytic anemia due to erythrophagocytosis by histiocytes. *Ann Intern Med, 63:* 666, 1965.

160. Maldonado, J. E. and Hanlon, D. G.: Monocytosis: a current appraisal. *Mayo Clin Proc, 40:* 248, 1965.

161. Mallory, F. B.: A histological study of typhoid fever. *J Exptl Med, 3:* 611, 1968.

162. Mann, W. N.: Monocytic leukaemia. *Guy's Hosp Rep, 85:* 178, 1935.

163. Marchal, G.; Lemoine, J. and Block-Michel, R.: Leucemie chronique à monocytes, sans splenomegalie, ni adenomegalie. *Sang, 8:* 694, 1934.

164. Marin-Padilla, M.; Fahimi, H. D. and Moloney, W. C.: Leukemic reticulum cell sarcoma (reticulum cell sarcoma terminating in acute leukemia). *Am J Clin Pathol, 41:* 402, 1964.

165. Mathé, G.; Gerard-Marchant, R.; Texier, J. L.; Schlumberger, J. R.; Berumen, L. and Paintrand, M.: The two varieties of lymphoid tissue "reticulosarcomas," histiocytic and histioblastic types. *Br J Cancer, 24:* 687, 1970.

166. Maximow, A. A.: Weiteres ueber Entstehung, Struktur und Veraenderungen des Farbengewebes. *Beitr Z Pathol Ant, 34:* 153, 1903.

167. ————: Development of non-granular leukocytes (lymphocytes) and monocytes into polyblasts (macrophages) and fibroblasts *in vitro. Proc Soc Exp Biol Med, 24:* 570, 1927.

168. ————: Cultures of blood leukocyte from lymphocyte and monocyte to connective tissue. *Arch Exp Zell Forsch, 5:* 169, 1928.

169. ————: The macrophages or histiocytes. In E. V. Cowdrey (Ed.): *Special Cytology.* New York, P. B. Hoeber, 1932, p. 427.

170. McAlpine, K. P.: A case of polycythemia rubra vera with leukemic blood picture. *JAMA, 92:* 1825, 1929.

171. McDuffie, N. G.: Nuclear blebs in human leukaemic cells. *Nature, 214:* 1341, 1967.

172. McJunkin, F. A.: The origin of the phagocytic mononuclear cells of the peripheral blood. *Am J Anat, 25:* 27, 1919.

173. ————: The identification of two types of mononuclear phagocytes in the peripheral blood of rabbits. *Proc Soc Exp Biol Med, 23:* 64, 1925.

174. ————: The origin of the mononuclear phagocytes of peritoneal exudates. *Am J Pathol, 1:* 304, 1925.

175. ————: The identification of three types of mononuclear phagocytes in the peripheral blood. *Arch Intern Med, 35:* 799, 1925.

176. ————: The large mononuclear and the transitional leukocyte of human blood. *J Lab Clin Med, 12:* 71, 1926.

177. McLean, J. A.: Supravital staining of the large mononuclear cells in infectious mononucleosis and the acute leuch-anemias with particular reference to their origin in the former disease. *Med J Aust, 2:* 734, 1929.

178. Meacham, G. C. and Weisberger, A. S.: Early atypical manifestations of leukemia. *Ann Intern Med, 41:* 780, 1954.

179. Medford, F. E.: Histiocytic medullary reticulosis: report of cases. *Arch Intern Med, 116:* 589, 1965.

180. Medlar, E. M.: An evaluation of the leukocytic reaction in the blood as found in cases of tuberculosis. *Am Rev Tuberc, 20:* 312, 1929.

181. ————: Further studies on the pathological significance of the leucocytic reaction in tuberculosis. *Am Rev Tuberc, 31:* 621, 1935.

182. Mercer, S. T.: Preliminary observations on human blood in early syphilis by the supravital method. *Proc Soc Exp Biol Med, 28:* 1033, 1931.

183. ————: The dermatosis of monocytic leukemia. *Arch Dermatol, 31:* 615, 1935.

184. Merklen, P. and Wolf, M.: Monocytes-monocytoses. Leucémies à monocytes. *La Presse Med, 35:* 145, 1927.

185. ———— and Wolf, M.: Leucémies à monocytes. *Rev Med, 45:* 153, 1928.

186. Metchnikoff, E.: *Lectures on the Comparative Pathology of Inflammation.* New York, Dover Publication, 1968.

187. Mitchell, L. A.: Malignant monoblastoma: a variant of monocytic leukemia. *Ann Intern Med, 8:* 1387, 1935.

188. Minot, G. R. and Smith, L. W.: The blood in tetrachlorethane poisoning. *Arch Intern Med, 28:* 687, 1921.

189. Mitus, W. J.; Mednicoff, I. B.; Witrels, B. and Dameshek, W.: Neoplastic lymphoid

reticulum cells in the peripheral blood: a histochemical study. *Blood, 17:* 206, 1961.

190. Mori, Y. and Lennert, K.: *Electron Microscopic Atlas of Lymph Node Cytology and Pathology.* Berlin, Springer-Verlag, 1969.

191. Mosier, D. E.: Cell interactions in the primary immune response *in vitro*: a requirement for specific cell clusters. *J Exp Med, 129:* 351, 1969.

192. Munger, M. and Huddleson, I. F.: A preliminary report of the blood picture in brucellosis. *J Lab Clin Med, 24:* 617, 1939.

193. Murray, E. G. P.; Webb, R. A. and Swaun, M. B. R.: A disease of rabbits characterized by a large mononuclear leukocytosis caused by a hitherto undescribed bacillis bacteria monocytogenes. *J Pathol Bacteriol, 29:* 407, 1926.

194. Murthy, M. S. N. and Von Haam, E.: The occurrence of the sex chromatin in white blood cells of young adults. *Am J Clin Pathol, 30:* 216, 1958.

195. Naegeli, O.: Ueber rothes Knochemark und Myeloblasten. *Deutsch Med Wochensch, 26:* 287, 1900.

196. ———: Das Blut. In L. Aschoff: *Pathologische Anatomie,* 1923, vol. 2, p. 156.

197. ———: *Blutkrankleiten und Blutdiagnostik.* Berlin, Verlag von Julius Springer, 1931.

198. ———: *Differential Diagnosis in Internal Medicine.* Chicago, S. B. DeBour, 1940.

199. Natelson, E. A.; Lynch, E. C. and Hettig, R. A.: Histiocytic medullary reticulosis. The role of phagocytosis in pancytopenia. *Arch Intern Med, 122:* 223, 1968.

200. Nowell, P. C.: Prognostic value of marrow chromosome studies in human "preleukemia." *Arch Pathol, 80:* 205, 1965.

201. Oberling, C.: Les réticulosarcomas et les réticuloendotheliosarcomes de la molle osseuse (sarcomes d'Ewing). *Bull Assn Franc Cancer, 17:* 259, 1928.

202. Ohara, K.; Fried, J.; Dowling, M. D., Jr.; Bittar, E. S. and Clarkson, B. D.: Studies of cellular proliferation in human leukemia. VII—Cytokinetic behavior of neoplastic cells in a patient with reticulum cell sarcoma in a leukemic phase. *Cancer, 28:* 862, 1971.

203. Orr, J. W.: Monocytic leukemia. *Lancet, I:* 403, 1933.

204. Osgood, C. W. and Lyght, C. E.: Monocytic leucemia with report of two cases. *J Lab Clin Med, 18:* 612, 1932.

205. Osgood, E. E.: Monocytic leukemia. *Arch Intern Med, 59:* 931, 1937.

206. Osserman, E. F. and Lawlor, D. P.: Serum and urinary lysozyme (muramidase) in monocytic and myelomonocytic leukemia. *J Exp Med, 124:* 921, 1966.

207. Ottander, O.: Hochgradige Endotheliose im Blut bei endocarditis lenta. *Acta Med Scand, 63:* 336, 1926.

208. Pappenheim, A. and Ferrata, A.: Ueber die verschiedenen lymphoiden Zellformen des normalen und pathologischen Blutes. *Folia Haematol, 10:* 78, 1910.

209. ———: Ueber verschiedenen Typen von Lymphozyten und Monozyten, zum Teil im scheinbar normalen Blut. *Folia Haematol, 12:* 26, 1911.

210. Patella, V.: La genesi endoteliale dei monociti, delle forme passaggio il dei considetti linfociti del sangue. *Haematologica, 4:* 59, 1933.

211. Pepper, O. H. P.: The hematology of subacute bacterial streptococcus viridans endocarditis. *JAMA, 89:* 1377, 1927.

212. Persaud, V. and Wood, J. K.: Histiocytic medullary reticulosis: a report of the first case in Jamaica. *Am J Clin Pathol, 4:* 396, 1967.

213. Petrakis, N. L.; Davis, N. and Lucia, S. P.: The *in vitro* differentiation of human

leukocytes into histiocytes, fibroblasts, and fat cells in subcutaneous diffusion chambers. *Blood, 17:* 109, 1961.

214. Plenderleith, I. H.: Hairy cell leukemia. *Canad Med Assn J, 102:* 1056, 1970.
215. Pretlow, T. G.: Chronic monocytic dyscrasia culminating in acute leukemia. *Am J Med, 46:* 130, 1969.
216. Ranvier, L.: Des clasmatocytes. *Arch Anat Microsc Morphol Exp, 3:* 123, 1899.
217. Rappaport, H.: *Tumors of the hematopoietic system. Armed Forces Inst Pathol,* 1966.
218. Rappoport, A. E. and Kugel, V. H.: Monocytic leukemia: case report illustrating variation in the clinical practice. *Blood, 2:* 332, 1947.
219. Rebuck, J. W.; Abraham, J. P. and Short, M.: Structural aspects of megakaryocytic function and lymphocyte relationships. In *Formation and Destruction of Blood Cells.* Philadelphia, J. B. Lippincott, 1970, p. 151.
220. Reeves, D. L.: A study of the *in vivo* and *in vitro* behavior of the monocytes of blood stream and connective tissue. *Bull Johns Hopkins Hosp, 55:* 245, 1934.
221. Reschad, H. and Schilling, V.: Ueber eine neue Leukaemie durch echte Uebergangs-formen (Splenozytenleukamie) und ihre Bedeutung fuer die Selbstaendigkeit dieser Zellen. *Muench Med Wochenschr, 60:* 198, 1913.
222. Reznikoff, P.: The etiologic importance of fatigue and the prognostic significance of monocytosis in neutropenia (agranulocytosis). *Am J Med Sci, 195:* 627, 1938.
223. Rezzesi, F. D.: La infezione da "bacterium monocytogenes" e i problemi del mono-cito. *Haematol, 14:* 239, 1933.
224. Rheingold, J. J.; Kaufman, R.; Adelson, F. and Lear, A.: Smouldering acute leukemia. *N Engl J Med, 268:* 812, 1963.
225. Richter, M. N.: The origin and development of monocytes in monocytic leukemia. *Arch Pathol, 1:* 841, 1926.
226. Riley, J. A. and Robins, G. M.: Leukemoid reaction due to mixed malarial infection: report of a case. *Blood, 4:* 283, 1949.
227. Rinehart, J. F.: The stem cell of the monocyte. *Arch Pathol, 13:* 889, 1932.
228. Ritchie, G. and Meyer, O. O.: Reticuloendotheliosis. *Arch Pathol, 22:* 729, 1936.
229. Robb-Smith, A. H. T.: Reticulosis and reticulosarcoma: histological classification. *J Pathol Bacteriol, 47:* 457, 1938.
230. Rohr, K.: *Das Menschliche Knochenmark.* Stuttgart, Georg Thieme Verlag, 1960.
231. Rohkramer, H.: Zur Klinik und Pathologie der aleukaemischen System-Reticulose. *Z Klin Med, 146:* 310, 1950.
232. Rosenthal, D. S. and Moloney, W. C.: The treatment of acute granulocytic leukemia in adults. *N Engl J Med, 286:* 1176, 1972.
233. Rosenthal, N.: Some atypical cases of leukemia. *Med Clin North Am, 4:* 1607, 1921.
234. ———— and Abel, H. A.: The significance of the monocytes in agranulocytosis. *Am J Clin Pathol, 6:* 205, 1936.
235. Rozenszajn, L.; Leibovich, M. and Shoham, D.: The esterase activity in megalo-blasts, leukemic and normal hemopoietic cells. *Br J Haematol, 14:* 605, 1968.
236. Roulet, F.: Das primaere Retothelsarkom der Lymphknoten. *Virchows Arch, 277:* 15, 1930.
237. ————: Weitere Beitraege zur Kenntnis des Retothelsarkoms der Lymphknoten und anderer lymphoiden Organe. *Virchows Arch, 286:* 702, 1932.
238. Rowley, J. D.; Blaisdell, R. K. and Jacobson, L. O.: Chromosome studies in pre-leukemia. I. Aneuploidy of group C chromosomes in three patients. *Blood, 27:* 782, 1966.

239. Rowley, M. W.: A fatal anemia with enormous numbers of circulating phagocytes. *J Exp Med, 10:* 786, 1908.

240. Rubin, A. D.; Douglas, S. D.; Chessin, L. N.; Glade, R. R. and Dameshek, W.: Chronic reticulolymphocytic leukemia: reclassification of 'leukemic reticulo-endotheliosis' through functional characterization of the circulating mononuclear cells. *Am. J Med, 47:* 149, 1969.

241. Ryder, R. J. W.: Chronic monocytic leukemia. *Blut, 14:* 47, 1966.

242. Saarni, M. I. and Linman, J. W.: Myelomonocytic leukemia: disorderly proliferation of all marrow cells. *Cancer, 27:* 1221, 1971.

243. Sabin, F. R.: Studies of living human blood-cells. *Bull Johns Hopkins Hosp, 34:* 217, 1923.

244. ———; Doan, C. A. and Cunningham, R. S.: The separation of the phagocytic cells of the peritoneal exudate into two distinct types. *Proc Soc Exp Biol Med, 21:* 330, 1924.

245. ———; Austrian, C. R.; Cunningham, R. S. and Doan, C. A.: Studies on the maturation of myeloblasts into myelocytes and on amitotic cell division in the peripheral blood in subacute myeloblastic leukemia. *J Exp Med, 40:* 845, 1924.

246. ———; Doan, C. A. and Cunningham, R. S.: The discrimination of two types of phagocytic cells in the connective tissue by the supravital technique. *Carneg Cont Emb, 16:* 125, 1925.

247. ———: Cellular reactions to fractions isolated from tubercle bacilli. *Phys Rev, 12:* 141, 1932.

248. Sampson, J. J.; Kerr, W. J. and Simpson, M. E.: A study of macrophages. *Arch Intern Med, 31:* 830, 1923.

249. Schilling, V.: Ueber hochgradige Monozytosen mit Makrophagen bei endocarditis ulcerosa und ueber die Herkunft der ar. mononuklearen. *Z Klin Med, 88:* 377, 1919.

250. ———: *Das Blutbild und Seine Klinische Verwertung.* Jena, G. Fisher, 1924.

251. ———: Der Monozyt in trialistischer Auffassung und seine Bedeutung im Krankheitsbilde. *Med Klin, 22:* 536, 1926.

252. ———: *The Blood Picture and Its Clinical Significance.* St. Louis, C. V. Mosby, 1929.

253. Schilling-Torgau, V.: *Das Blutbild.* Jena, Fisher, 1912.

254. Schmalzl, F. and Braunsteiner, H.: Cytochemische Darstellung von Esteraseaktivitaet in Blut—und Knochenmarkzellen. *Klin Wochenschr, 46:* 642, 1968.

255. ——— and Braunsteiner, M.: On the origin of monocytes. *Acta Haematol, 39:* 177, 1968.

256. ———; Huber, H.; Asamer, H.; Abbrederis, K. and Braunsteiner, H.: Cytochemical and immunohistological investigation on the source and the functional changes of mononuclear cells in skin window exudates. *Blood, 34:* 129, 1969.

257. ——— and Braunsteiner, H.: The cytochemistry of monocytes and macrophages. *Ser Haematol, 3:* 93, 1970.

258. Schnitzer, B. and Kass, L.: Refractory sideroblastic anemia (chronic erythremic myelosis). *Am J Clin Pathol,* (in press).

259. ——— and Kaas, L.: Leukemic phase of reticulum cell sarcoma (histiocytic lymphoma). A clinicopathologic and ultrastructural study. *Cancer, 31:* 547, 1973.

260. Schoenberg, M. D.; Mumaro, V. R.; Moore, R. D. and Weisberger, A. S.: Cytoplasmic interaction between macrophages and lymphocytic cells in antibody synthesis. *Science, 143:* 964, 1964.

261. Scholnik, A. and Kass, L.: Direct cytochemical demonstration of lysozyme in a variety of tissues. *J Histochem Cytochem, 21:* 65, 1973.

262. Schrek, R. and Donnelly, W. J.: "Hairy" cells in blood in lymphoreticular neoplastic disease and flagellated cells in normal lymph nodes. *Blood, 27:* 199, 1966.

263. Schwartz, S. O. and Critchlow, J.: Erythremic myelosis (DiGuglielmo's disease). Critical review with report of four cases and comments on erythroleukemia. *Blood, 7:* 765, 1952.

264. Scott, R. and Robb-Smith, A. H. T.: The progressive hyperplasias of the reticuloendothelial system. *St. Barts Hosp Rep, 69:* 143, 1936.

265. ———— and Robb-Smith, A. H. T.: Histiocytic medullary reticulosis. *Lancet, 237:* 194, 1939.

266. Scott, R. B.; Ellison, R. R. and Ley, A. B.: A clinical study of twenty cases of erythroleukemia (DiGuglielmo syndrome). *Am J Med, 37:* 162, 1964.

267. Sega, A. and Brustolon, D. A.: Leucemia monocitica o reticuloendoteliosi leucemica? *Haematol, 10:* 471, 1929.

268. Semsroth, K.: Leukemic reticuloendotheliosis, its relation to the blood picture of lymphatic leukemia. *Folia Haematol, 52:* 132, 1934.

269. Serck-Hanssen, A. and Purchit, G. P.: Histiocytic medullary reticulosis. Report of 14 cases from Uganda. *Br J Cancer, 22:* 506, 1968.

270. Sézary, A. and Bouvrain, Y.: Erythrodermie avec presence de cellules monstreuses dans la dermie et le sang circulant. *Bull Soc Franc Dermatol Syphiligr, 45:* 254, 1938.

271. ————: Une nouvelle reticulose cutaneé. *Ann Dermatol Syphiligr, 9:* 5, 1949.

272. Silhol, J. and Rouslacroix, A.: Sarcome d'origine ganglionaire à disposition strictement peritheliale (tumeur de l'aisselle). *Bull Assn Etude Cancer, 13:* 739, 1924.

273. Simpson, M. E.: The experimental production of macrophages in the circulating blood. *J Med Res, 43:* 77, 1922.

274. ————: Vital staining of human and mammalian blood with special reference to the separation of the monocytes. *Anat Rec, 23:* 37, 1922. (abstr.)

275. Sinn, C. M. and Dick, F. W.: Monocytic leukemia. *Am J Med, 20:* 588, 1956.

276. Stasney, J. and Downey, H.: Subacute lymphatic leukemia. *Am J Pathol, 11:* 113, 1935.

277. Steiner, M.; Baldini, M. and Dameshek, W.: Heme synthesis defect in "refractory" anemias with ineffective erythropoiesis. *Blood, 22:* 810, 1963.

278. Sternberger, L. A.; Osserman, E. F. and Seligman, A. M.: Lysozyme and fibrinogen in normal and leukemic blood cells: a quantitative electron microscopic and immunochemical study. *Johns Hopkins Med J, 126:* 188, 1970.

279. Stone, G. E. and Redmond, A. J.: Leukopenic infectious monocytosis: report of a case closely simulating acute monocytic leukemia. *Am J Med, 34:* 541, 1963.

280. Sutton, J. S. and Weiss, L.: Transformation of monocytes in tissue culture into macrophages, epithelioid cells and multinucleated giant cells. *J Cell Biol, 28:* 303, 1966.

281. Sydenstricker, V. P. and Phizini, T. B.: Acute monocytic leukemia: a case with partial autopsy. *Am J Med Sci, 184:* 770, 1932.

282. Tanaka, Y.: Fibrillar structure in cells of blood-forming organs. *J Nat Cancer Inst, 33:* 467, 1964.

283. Thomas, C. C.: Sarcoidosis. *Arch Dermatol Syphilol, 47:* 58, 1943.

284. Tompkins, E. H.: The response of monocytes to adrenal cortical extract. *J Lab Clin Med, 39:* 365, 1952.

285. ———: The monocyte. *Ann N Y Acad Sci, 59:* 732, 1953.

286. Trubowitz, S.; Masek, B. and Frasca, J. M.: Leukemic reticuloendotheliosis. *Blood, 38:* 288, 1971.

287. Vaithianathan, T.; Bolonik, S. J. and Gruhn, J. G.: Leukemic reticuloendotheliosis. *Am J Clin Pathol, 38:* 605, 1962.

288. ———; Fishkin, S. and Gruhan, J. G.: Histiocytic medullary reticulosis. *Am J Clin Pathol, 47:* 160, 1967.

289. Van den Ende, M.; Harries, E. H. R.; Stuart-Harris, C. H.; Steigman, A. J. and Cruickshank, R.: Laboratory infections with murine typhus. *Lancet, 1:* 328, 1943.

290. Van Furth, R. and Cohn, A. A.: The origin and kinetics of mononuclear phago-cytes. *J Exp Med, 128:* 415, 1968.

291. ———; Hirsch, J. F. and Fedorko, M. E.: Morphology and peroxidase cytochem-istry of mouse promonocytes, monocytes and macrophages. *J Exp Med, 132:* 794, 1970.

292. Van Nuys, F.: An extraordinary blood. *Boston Med Surg J, 156:* 390, 1907.

293. Verloop, M. C.; Panders, J. T.; Ploem, J. E. and Bos, C. C.: Sideroachrestic anaemias. *Series Haematol, 1:* 76, 1965.

294. Volkman, A. and Gowans, J. L.: The origin of macrophages from bone marrow in rats. *Br J Exp Pathol, 46:* 62, 1965.

295. ———: The origin and turnover of mononuclear cells in peritoneal exudates in rats. *J Exp Med, 124:* 241, 1966.

296. Vilter, R. W.; Will, J. J. and Jarrold, T.: Refractory anemia with hyperplastic bone marrow (aregenerative anemia). *Sem Hematol, 4:* 175, 1967.

297. Wainwright, C. W. and Duff, G. L.: Monocytic leukemia. *Bull Johns Hopkins Hosp, 58:* 267, 1936.

298. Watkins, C. H. and Hall, B. E.: Monocytic leukemia of the Naegeli and Schilling types. *Am J Clin Pathol, 10:* 387, 1940.

299. Whitby, L. and Christie, J.: Monocytic leukemia. *Lancet, 1:* 80, 1935.

300. Whitelaw, D. M.: The intravascular life span of monocytes. *Blood, 28:* 455, 1966.

301. Wile, U. J.; Isaacs, R. and Knerler, C. W.: The blood cells in early syphilis. *Am J Syph Gonorr Ven Dis, 25:* 133, 1941.

302. Willcox, D. R. C.: Hemolytic anaemia and reticulosis. *Br Med J, 1:* 1322, 1952.

303. Williams, M. J.: Myleoblastic leukemia preceded by prolonged hematologic dis-order. *Blood, 10:* 502, 1955.

304. Wintrobe, M. M. and Mitchell, D. M.: Atypical manifestations of leukemia. *Q J Med, 33:* 67, 1940.

305. Wiseman, B. K.: The origin of the white blood cells. *JAMA, 103:* 1524, 1934.

306. Witts, L. J. and Webb, R. A.: The monocytes of the rabbit in *B. monocytogenes* infection: a study of their staining reactions and histogenesis. *J Pathol Bacteriol, 30:* 687, 1927.

307. Yam, L. T.; Li, C. Y. and Crosby, W. H.: Cytochemical identification of mono-cytes and granulocytes. *Am J Clin Pathol, 55:* 283, 1971.

308. ———; Li, C. Y. and Lam, K. W.: Tartrate-resistant acid phosphatase isoenzyme in the reticulum cells of leukemic reticuloendotheliosis. *N Engl J Med, 284:* 357, 1971.

309. Yoshida, T.; Benacerraf, B.; McCluskey, R. T. and Vassalli, P. J.: The effects of intravenous antigen on circulating monocytes in animals with delayed hyper-sensitivity. *J Immunol, 102:* 800, 1969.

310. Youman, J. D.; Saarni, M. and Linman, J. W.: Diagnostic value of muramidase (lysozyme) in acute leukemia and preleukemia. *Mayo Clin Proc, 45:* 219, 1970.

311. Zak, F. G. and Rubin, E.: Histiocytic medullary reticulosis. *Am J Med, 31:* 813, 1961.
312. Zeffren, J. L. and Ultmann, J. E.: Reticulum cell sarcoma terminating in acute leukemia. *Blood, 15:* 277, 1960.

INDEX